Legal Disclaimer:

The following disclaimer is essential to be acknowledged before engaging with any material provided within this intermittent fasting book:

1. **Medical Consultation:** The content presented in this book is intended for informational purposes only. It is not intended to be a substitute for professional medical advice, diagnosis, or treatment. Before commencing any intermittent fasting regimen or making significant changes to your dietary habits, it is imperative to consult with a qualified healthcare professional or physician, especially if you have any pre-existing medical conditions or concerns regarding your health.

2. **Individualized Results:** Results obtained from intermittent fasting can vary significantly from person to person. Factors such as age, gender, genetics, medical history, lifestyle, and adherence to the program can all influence outcomes. The information provided in this book does not guarantee specific results and should not be construed as such. Individual experiences may differ, and success with intermittent fasting is not universal.

3. **Not a Substitute for Professional Advice:** The author of this book is not a medical professional or registered dietitian. While every effort has been made to ensure the accuracy and completeness of the information provided, the author cannot guarantee its applicability or relevance to every individual. Readers are encouraged to seek personalized advice from qualified professionals regarding their specific health and dietary needs.

4. **Assumption of Risk:** Engaging in intermittent fasting involves inherent risks, including but not limited to potential changes in metabolic function, fluctuations in blood sugar levels, and the possibility of adverse reactions. By choosing to implement any recommendations or strategies outlined in this book, readers assume full responsibility for their actions and any associated risks. The author disclaim liability for any damages, losses, or injuries arising directly or indirectly from the use or application of information contained herein.

5. **Accuracy of Information:** While every effort has been made to ensure the accuracy and reliability of the information presented in this book, the author make no representations or warranties, express or implied, regarding the completeness, suitability, or validity of any information provided. Readers are encouraged to verify any information obtained from this book with other reputable sources and to exercise caution when interpreting and applying dietary advice.

Contents

Introduction

"The greatest wealth is health."

Virgil

In a world filled with endless diet trends and fitness crazes, the discovery that intermittent fasting (IF) can dramatically improve the health of women over 50 is a beacon of hope and surprise. This book addresses the urgent need to challenge common misconceptions surrounding aging, hormonal balance, and weight management. By peeling away the layers of generic dietary advice, we uncover a less-traveled yet scientifically sound path specifically tailored to the unique needs of women approaching the golden era of their lives.

This guide is dedicated to demystifying IF for women over 50 by exploring science-based facts. These facts debunk myths and establish a solid foundation for an enlightening and life-changing fasting journey. Unlike other guides on IF, this book carves out a niche by focusing precisely on the needs and challenges faced by women over 50. We have created a simplified, empowering narrative with scientific research and practical advice.

Readers can expect numerous benefits from embracing the strategies outlined in this book. The benefits of improved metabolic health and weight loss to enhanced mental clarity and better hormonal balance are profound and firmly supported by science. This book will guide you through the maze of misinformation, devoid of medical jargon, and make complex scientific concepts accessible.

This book offers a comprehensive roadmap, beginning with understanding IF and its interaction with menopause. It then delves into tailored nutrition and exercise strategies, concluding with a guide to living the IF lifestyle. This structure aims to inform and engage you as an active participant in your health journey. Keeping an open mind, experimenting with the discussed strategies, and even documenting your fasting experience in a journal are highly encouraged.

The journey with intermittent fasting (IF), particularly its significant advantages for women over 50, has been enlightening and profoundly motivating. Although this introduction doesn't explore an individual biography, it's important to emphasize that this book is grounded in real-life experiences and thorough scientific research. It serves as an educational tool and an encouragement to take steps towards improving health through a transformative journey.

As you flip through these pages, remember that this journey you're embarking on is so much more than shedding weight – it's a pledge to a healthier, more radiant you as you embrace your 50s and beyond. This is your invitation to enter a new empowerment, health, and vitality era. Let's start this beautiful chapter together.

Chapter 1

The Basics of Intermittent Fasting

"To keep the body in good health is a duty... otherwise we shall not be able to keep our mind strong and clear."

Buddha

You've heard about this intermittent fasting thing, also known as IF, and you're curious if it's right for you, especially as a woman over 50. Well, you're in the right place! In this chapter, we will break down the basics of IF explicitly tailored for women like us who are navigating the golden years. We'll explore what IF is all about, how it can benefit women over 50, and some practical tips to get started on your fasting journey. So, let's dive in and uncover the secrets to feeling your best.

What is IF and How It Works

So, what exactly is IF? Well, it's not your typical diet. Instead of focusing on what you eat, it's all about when you eat. It involves cycling between periods of eating and fasting. This concept isn't new—it's been around for ages, driven by necessity and religious practices, and now it's gaining popularity for its health benefits.

There are different ways to do IF, but three methods stand out: the 16/8 method, the 5:2 method, and the eat-stop-eat plan. With the 16/8 method, you fast for 16 hours a day and eat during an 8-hour window. It's simple and can easily fit into your daily routine. The 5:2 method lets you usually eat five days a week and restricts your calorie intake to about 500-600 calories on the other two days. And then there's the eat-stop-eat plan, where you do 24-hour fasts once or twice a week. Each method offers flexibility, so you can choose what works best for you and your lifestyle.

But IF isn't just about weight loss—it goes much deeper. It triggers some fantastic changes in your body's cells and metabolism. One of the biggies is autophagy, which is your body's way of cleaning out damaged cells and regenerating new ones. This process helps reduce inflammation and fight off diseases. Plus, IF improves insulin sensitivity, which is crucial for managing weight and reducing the risk of diabetes. By tweaking hormone levels, fasting helps your body use fat stores for energy more efficiently, aiding in weight loss and overall metabolic health.

And get this—IF isn't just good for your body; it's excellent for your brain, too! Studies show it can boost brain health, improve cognitive function, and even lower the risk of neurodegenerative diseases. This is partly because fasting increases brain-derived neurotrophic factor (BDNF) levels, a protein that supports neuron survival and brain function.

IF can also reduce inflammation and oxidative stress, lowering one's risk of chronic diseases like heart disease, cancer, and Alzheimer's. So yeah, it's powerful stuff!

In a nutshell, IF is a versatile and practical way to improve your health and well-being, especially for women over 50 facing unique health challenges. Its different methods can fit into anyone's lifestyle, offering a feasible and attractive option for those looking to boost their health. Its profound effects on cellular mechanisms and its ability to go beyond weight loss make IF valuable in pursuing a long and vibrant life. So, if you're curious about exploring this eating pattern, you're not alone. A whole community of women is discovering its benefits and embracing it on their journey to better health!

Autophagy: Turning the Body's Self-Cleansing Mode On

Let's talk about autophagy—a fascinating process like hitting the reset button for your body's cells. It is a natural cleanup crew within your body. The word itself comes from Greek and means "self-eating." Pretty cool, right? Essentially, autophagy is your body's way of cleaning out damaged cells and making room for fresh, healthy ones. It's like a deep cleanse for your cells, helping to keep them in tip-top shape.

Now, why is autophagy so essential, especially for women over 50? This process can help slow aging, boost cellular health, and even balance hormones. And guess what? IF is a powerful way to kickstart autophagy into high gear.

Here's how it works: when you fast, your body's energy levels drop, signaling to your cells that it's time to tidy up shop. This prompts them to start breaking down and recycling damaged components, like taking out the trash. By doing this, your cells stay healthy and efficient, which benefits your overall health.

For women going through menopause, the perks of enhanced autophagy are especially exciting. Not only can it help improve the health of your skin by clearing out damaged cells, but it also plays a crucial role in preventing diseases. By eliminating those old, worn-out cells, autophagy reduces the risk of age-related illnesses like cancer, Alzheimer's, and metabolic disorders. Plus, it helps keep your hormones in check by supporting the organs responsible for hormone production.

Now, if you want to make the most of autophagy through IF, here are some tips to keep in mind:

- Start slow and gradually increase your fasting periods as your body gets used to it.

- Stay hydrated during fasting periods to help flush out toxins and debris from your cells.

- Get moving! Exercise, especially during fasting windows, can boost the autophagy response.

- Make sure you're getting enough sleep, as this is when your body does most of its repair work, including autophagy.

- Eat nutrient-rich foods during your eating windows to support cellular health and maximize the benefits of autophagy.

- Practice mindfulness and stress reduction techniques to create a balanced internal environment that supports autophagy.

By incorporating these strategies into your IF routine, you can tap into the rejuvenating power of autophagy and promote vitality and health as you age. It's all about giving your cells the TLC they need to keep you feeling your best!

Insulin Sensitivity: How it Affects Your Weight and Health

Insulin sensitivity refers to your body's ability to utilize energy effectively. It lowers your blood sugar levels after eating by allowing glucose to enter your cells, providing the energy your body needs to function correctly. Your body's energy language is fluent when everything works as it should. However, if your cells become less responsive to insulin, it can lead to insulin resistance, which is a severe health issue that can result in type 2 diabetes.

Now, things get interesting here, especially for women hitting their 50s. Menopause can mess with this whole insulin sensitivity thing. As estrogen levels drop, insulin resistance can get worse, making it more challenging to manage your weight and keep your blood sugar levels stable. Plus, it can cause fat to pile up around your belly, making weight management even trickier.

But fear not! There's a powerful tool in your toolbox: IF. Research shows that fasting can help lower insulin levels, prompting your body to burn fat for energy instead of relying on glucose. This helps with weight loss and improves insulin sensitivity by easing the demand for insulin in your body. Fasting can dial down inflammation and other markers of metabolic issues like blood sugar levels and cholesterol.

So, how can you tailor IF to boost your insulin health? Here are some tips:

Start slow and gradually increase as you get used to it. Shorter fasts during the day work better for some people.

When you eat, focus on whole foods packed with fiber, healthy fats, and lean proteins. It helps slow down sugar absorption, keeping your blood sugar and insulin levels steady.

Be mindful of the types and amounts of carbs you eat. Aim for complex carbs with a low glycemic index to prevent spikes in blood sugar.

Get moving! Regular exercise, especially strength training, and aerobic workouts can improve your muscles' ability to use glucose, improving insulin sensitivity.

Drink up! Staying hydrated is vital for keeping your blood sugar levels in check.

Prioritize sleep and stress management. Aim for 7-9 hours of quality sleep each night and find ways to relax and destress, like meditation or yoga.

By following these strategies, you can customize your IF plan to support your insulin health, making weight management easier and lowering your risk of metabolic diseases. It's all about finding a balance that works for you and keeps you feeling your best as you journey into your 50s and beyond.

Menopause: How Hormonal Shifts Mess with Your Metabolism

Understanding how menopause and metabolism interact can help explain why managing weight can become trickier as one enters one's 50s and beyond.

First off, what exactly happens during menopause? Well, it's a significant change in your body's hormonal balance. One of the main things that occurs is a drop in estrogen levels. Estrogen does more than regulate your reproductive system—it also significantly impacts your metabolism, the process by which your body converts food into energy.

When estrogen levels go down, it can affect where your body stores fat. You might notice more fat accumulating around your abdomen, which can be frustrating. Plus, the hormonal changes can make you tired more often, making it harder to stay active and burn calories.

But that's not all. As we get older, our metabolism naturally slows down. This happens for a few reasons. One is the decrease in basal metabolic rate (BMR), which is how much energy your body uses when you're at rest. Another factor is the loss of muscle mass, a condition known as sarcopenia. Muscles play a crucial role in keeping your metabolism humming, so when you lose muscle, your metabolism can slow down even more.

So, what does all this mean for managing your weight? It means your body might need fewer calories than it used to maintain its essential functions. That means you might need to adjust your diet and exercise routine accordingly to prevent weight gain.

Understanding how menopause and metabolism are connected can help you make informed choices about caring for your body as you age. It's all about finding a balance for you and your changing needs.

Imagine this: By tweaking when you eat, IF can help your body manage blood sugar levels better, reducing the chance of storing extra fat. It's pretty cool, right?

Not only that, but IF encourages your body to switch from using glucose (sugar) as its primary energy source to burning fat. This happens because when you fast for a while, your body starts tapping into its fat stores for fuel.

But wait, there's more! IF can also bump up human growth hormone levels (HGH). This hormone is like a superhero—it helps your body burn fat and build muscle. And since losing muscle becomes more common as we age, especially during menopause, anything that prevents that loss is a win in my book!

Now, if you're a woman going through menopause, you might be wondering how to tailor IF to fit your unique hormonal changes. Here are some tips just for you:

First, pick a fasting schedule that works with your body's natural rhythms. Closing your eating window earlier in the evening can help regulate blood sugar levels and improve sleep—a win-win!

When you eat, focus on nutrient-packed foods rich in phytoestrogens, fiber, and omega-3 fatty acids. These goodies can help keep your hormones happy and your metabolism humming.

Protein is your friend, especially when keeping your muscles strong. So, make sure to include plenty of protein-rich foods in your meals during your eating windows.

And most importantly, listen to your body! Everyone's experience with menopause is different, so pay attention to how fasting makes you feel. If shorter fasts work better for you, go for it. And if fasting leaves you feeling drained, it's okay to tweak your schedule or skip it altogether.

By tailoring IF to fit your needs, you can tap into its incredible benefits and support your health during this exciting—and sometimes challenging—stage of life.

Addressing Common Menopausal Symptoms with IF

Menopause, huh? It's like going through your season with a mix of unexpected twists—hot flashes, restless nights, mood rollercoasters, and that pesky brain fog. But there's a silver lining: IF might be a friendly companion through this time. Let's dive into how tweaking when you eat could lend a hand during these changing times.

First off, those infamous hot flashes and night sweats can be a real nuisance. But here's a thought: Could you help dial down their frequency and intensity? It's linked to better insulin sensitivity and reduced inflammation, which can calm the hormonal storms causing those heat waves. Shedding a few extra pounds with IF might reduce hot flashes since body fat acts like a personal heater.

Now, onto the whole sleep saga. If counting sheep isn't cutting it anymore, IF could help. By balancing your blood sugar and encouraging your body to produce melatonin earlier (our sleep hormone), IF could help you catch those elusive Z's. Less food in the evening means more room for your body to wind down and slip into dreamland.

Let's remember the emotional and mental side of things. IF could be a beacon of hope for moodiness and foggy thinking. It boosts brain health, cuts inflammation, and might even improve gut health, which is surprisingly linked to mood and brain function. Combining IF with calming activities like meditation could help smooth out those emotional highs and lows.

Here's a quick word on eating right: while IF isn't all about what you eat, the "what" still matters. Menopause is a time to focus on what your body needs. Foods rich in phytoestrogens, calcium, vitamin D, and omega-3 fatty acids can be particularly supportive. And don't forget to keep hydrated and pack in the fiber—your body will thank you.

Menopause can be challenging, but with the flexible approach of IF, it can be a bit more manageable. The key is to time your meals to support your body's changing needs. Whether you want to reduce hot flashes, improve your sleep, boost your mood, or clear the fog, IF can help you customize your diet to suit your body's rhythm during this time. Remember that every woman's journey is unique, so it's all about finding what works best for you.

Customizing Your Fasting Window for Hormonal Health

Let's chat about tailoring your fasting schedule to nourish your hormonal health, especially during the rollercoaster ride that is menopause. It's like discovering a hidden doorway that leads to a more balanced you. During menopause, your body goes through a whirlwind of hormonal changes that can reduce your metabolism, mood, and energy levels. By syncing your eating and fasting times with these changes, you can soften some of menopause's rough edges. For example, fasting at night takes advantage of when your body naturally becomes less sensitive to insulin, which can help your blood sugar levels and may lead to better sleep.

Now, tuning into your body's cues is crucial here. Menopause isn't a one-size-fits-all event. What works for your friend might work better for you. If you're feeling more irritable or tired with a longer fast, it might be a nudge from your body to try a shorter fasting period or to eat a little earlier. Your body will give you feedback, and listening to it is critical to adjusting your fasting plan to lift you rather than drag you down.

Integrating fasting into your daily life can be tricky with all the juggling you do between work, family, and social life. It's about finding a rhythm that doesn't feel like you're sacrificing too much. Planning can make a world of difference. Do you have a social gathering coming up? Adjust your fasting window that day. Remember to chat about your fasting schedule with your loved ones; they will likely support you once they understand your goals. Packing nutritious meals for on-the-go and focusing on mindful eating when you sit down to eat can also help you seamlessly mesh your fasting with your life.

Think of fasting as a personal experiment. Start with something manageable, like a 12-hour fast, and then you can play around for more extended periods. Notice how your body and mood respond. Some might find a 14-hour fast is their happy place, balancing well with their lifestyle, while others might benefit more from pushing it to 16 hours. Remember, this is about finding what feels suitable for you.

When you're tweaking your fasting lengths, watch your menopausal symptoms and how they shift. A gradual approach is gentler on your body than drastic changes. And when breaking your fast, choosing a meal rich in proteins, healthy fats, and fiber can help keep your energy steady. Because our bodies and lives keep evolving, revisiting and refining your fasting plan is good practice.

Remember, navigating menopause and finding the best fasting routine is deeply personal. There's no universal solution, but by listening closely to your body and making thoughtful adjustments, IF can be a supportive ally through menopause and beyond.

How IF Can Improve Your Mind and Mood

Ever feel like your brain's stuck in a fog during menopause? You're not alone. But guess what? IF might be the trick to clear things up. When you fast, your body produces these little things called ketones, which are like super fuel for your brain. They help sharpen your focus and boost cognitive function, giving you more productive days and a newfound confidence in your mental abilities.

And speaking of mood swings, we all know how hormones can throw us for a loop during menopause. However, IF can help smooth out those ups and downs. By reducing inflammation and balancing out your hormones, fasting can lead to a more stable mood. Plus, you'll ride a steadier emotional wave when your body gets better at regulating insulin and stress hormones like cortisol.

Now, let's talk about the power of commitment. Adopting IF isn't just about changing your diet—it's a lifestyle shift. And as you stick to your fasting and eating schedule, you build resilience and discipline that spill over into other areas of your life. Whether sticking to a workout routine or managing your time more effectively, the discipline you cultivate through fasting can help you achieve your goals.

But it's not just about when you eat—it's also about how you eat. IF encourages you to be more mindful about your meals. Instead of mindlessly munching in front of the TV, you'll start planning and savoring your food. And when you only have a limited food window, you'll find yourself making healthier choices that nourish your body. Over time, this mindful approach can help you break free from emotional eating habits and develop a deeper appreciation for food as fuel.

So, if you're looking to clear the mental fog, stabilize your mood, and cultivate resilience and discipline—all while fostering a healthier relationship with food—IF might be the answer you've been searching for. Give it a try and see how it transforms not just your body but your mind and spirit, too!

How IF Can Help You Live Longer

Humans have been on a quest for longevity for centuries, and recent scientific studies have uncovered a potential key: IF. This approach to eating isn't just about cutting calories—it's about strategically timing our meals to promote optimal health and vitality as we age.

So, how is IF linked to longevity? Well, research tells us that it can profoundly impact our health span, the period of life spent in good health. By reducing oxidative stress and inflammation—two major players in the aging process—fasting helps preserve the integrity and function of our cells, setting the stage for a longer, healthier life.

But IF's benefits go even deeper, fundamentally influencing our cellular and hormonal systems. For example, fasting promotes autophagy, which cleanses damaged cells and stimulates cellular regeneration. It also boosts levels of human growth hormone (HGH), which helps maintain muscle mass, improve fat metabolism, and enhance physical performance. By improving insulin sensitivity and reducing inflammation, fasting can lower the risk of type 2 diabetes and other age-related diseases.

As we age, our bodies undergo changes that may affect how we respond to fasting. That's why it's crucial to adapt our fasting practices over time. We can tweak the length of fasting periods, pay more attention to our nutritional intake during eating windows, or incorporate gentler forms of fasting that don't put too much stress on the body. The key is to listen to our bodies and adjust how we feel.

And let's remember the preventive measures IF offers against age-related diseases. From heart disease and Alzheimer's to osteoporosis and cancer, fasting can help reduce the risk of these conditions by improving various risk factors and promoting overall health and well-being.

By incorporating IF into our lives, we're opening a promising pathway to living longer and healthier. By understanding the science behind fasting and its impact on longevity, we can make informed decisions about integrating this practice into our daily routine. It's not just about adding years to our lives but life to our years—ensuring that we can enjoy our later years with vitality, health, and happiness. So, let's embrace the power of IF and embark on a journey to a longer, healthier life together!

Debunking Myths: Separating IF Facts from Fiction

Let's clear up common misconceptions around IF for women over 50 amidst conflicting information.

Myth: IF Causes Muscle Loss

Reality: Contrary to popular belief, IF doesn't necessarily lead to muscle loss. It can improve hormone function, help with weight loss, and even boost muscle strength when combined with resistance training. During fasting, your body primarily burns fat for fuel, preserving muscle mass if you get enough protein during your eating windows.

Myth: IF Leads to Starvation Mode

Reality: IF can boost metabolism by increasing the norepinephrine hormone, which aids in burning body fat. The concept of starvation mode only comes into play when an individual undergoes extreme and prolonged calorie restriction, not during the controlled fasting periods typical of IF.

Myth: IF will worsen menopause symptoms

Reality: Some women find that IF helps with menopause symptoms like hot flashes. However, individual experiences vary.

Myth: IF is too challenging for older women

Reality: Many older women successfully incorporate it into their lifestyles. Starting with short fasting periods or consulting a healthcare provider can help it more manageable.

Addressing Fears About Fasting and Menopause Concern

Fear not! IF might help improve hormonal balance and reduce inflammation, potentially easing symptoms like hot flashes and mood swings. The key is finding a fasting approach that supports your body's natural rhythms without adding extra stress.

Concern: IF Could Mess with Hormonal Health. Good news! IF can enhance insulin sensitivity and reduce insulin levels, which are great for hormonal regulation. Choose nutrient-dense foods to support overall hormonal health during your eating windows.

Evidence-Based Benefits. IF offers more than just weight management perks; it's backed by science! Here are some evidence-based benefits, especially relevant for women over 50:

- **Improved Insulin Sensitivity:** IF helps regulate blood sugar, lowering the risk of type 2 diabetes.

- **Enhanced Brain Function:** Fasting boosts protein levels called BDNF, which supports cognitive health and may help fend off conditions like Alzheimer's.

- **Increased Longevity:** Animal studies suggest IF could extend lifespan by reducing oxidative stress and enhancing cellular repair.

- **Better Cardiovascular Health:** IF can lower blood pressure, improve cholesterol levels, and decrease the risk of heart disease by enhancing metabolic markers.

Consulting Healthcare Professionals. Before diving headfirst into IF, it's wise to consult with healthcare professionals, especially if you're new to it or have existing health concerns. Here's why:

- **Personalized Assessment:** To offer tailored guidance, your healthcare provider can evaluate your health status, medical history, and nutritional needs.

- **Addressing Existing Conditions:** For women with diabetes or heart disease, a healthcare professional can help design an IF plan that considers these factors, minimizing risks and maximizing benefits.

- **Monitoring Progress:** Regular check-ups allow your healthcare team to track how your body responds to IF and make any necessary adjustments to keep you healthy and feeling your best.

Embarking on an IF journey without professional guidance can pose risks, especially for women over 50 dealing with the unique challenges of menopause. With the proper support, IF can be a valuable addition to your lifestyle, promoting health and well-being without unnecessary stress or confusion.

Transitioning into IF: A Step-by-Step Guide

Transitioning into IF can feel like stepping into unknown territory, especially for women over 50 navigating the complexities of menopause. But fear not; with a thoughtful approach, you can ease into this lifestyle change, set achievable goals, track your progress, and find the support you need.

Starting Slow

Rushing into a strict fasting routine can leave you feeling overwhelmed and burnt out. Instead, take it slow. If you typically fast for 12 hours overnight, try extending that by an hour or two to start. This gradual adjustment gives your body time to adapt without feeling shocked, making the transition smoother and more manageable. As you become more comfortable, you can slowly increase your fasting window at the right pace.

Setting Realistic Goals

Goal setting is powerful, but it's essential to keep things realistic. When considering IF, align your goals with your current health, lifestyle, and any symptoms you manage. For instance, if improving insulin sensitivity is essential, gradually extend your overnight fasting period. If you're focusing on controlling weight gain during menopause, set a specific and sustainable fasting schedule that fits seamlessly into your daily routine without causing stress. Remember, goals can evolve as you progress.

Monitoring Progress and Adjusting

Keeping a close eye on your progress is vital. It's not just about what the scale says or how your waistline measures up. Pay attention to how you feel. Are you noticing increased energy levels? Are your menopausal symptoms becoming more manageable? Perhaps you've experienced improvements in sleep quality or mental clarity. Record these changes in a journal or a health-tracking app.

Also, be open to adjusting along the way. If you find that your current fasting schedule isn't working for you—maybe it's leaving you too hungry or not yielding the results you expected—don't hesitate to tweak it. This process is about finding what works best for your body and lifestyle.

Seeking Support

Embarking on an IF journey is personal, but that doesn't mean you have to go it alone. Support can make all the difference. Start by discussing your plans with a healthcare professional, especially if you have existing health concerns. They can offer tailored guidance and help you navigate any potential risks.

Community support is also invaluable. Joining a group or an online forum dedicated to IF can provide a wealth of shared experiences and advice. Here, you can find encouragement on tough days, celebrate your successes, and learn from others on a similar path. These platforms are great for troubleshooting common challenges and discovering practical tips to make your fasting experience more enjoyable and effective.

Transitioning to IF is a unique journey, influenced by individual health, lifestyle, and how your body responds to dietary changes. You can navigate this transition confidently and successfully by starting slowly, setting realistic goals, monitoring progress, and seeking support. Remember, the key to long-term success lies in sustainability and aligning your dietary choices with your body's needs and lifestyle. IF offers a flexible approach to improving health and well-being, adapting to your circumstances.

Fasting Safely: Avoiding Common Pitfalls and Missteps

Embarking on IF is a journey filled with discovery and adjustment, especially for women over 50 facing the intricacies of menopause. But fear not; with a mindful approach, you can sidestep common pitfalls and ensure a smooth transition into this lifestyle change. Let's dive in and explore how to fast safely while staying attuned to your body's needs at every step.

Recognizing Personal Limits

As you begin your IF journey, it's essential to tune in to your body's responses. Listen closely for signals that indicate when to proceed or pause your fasting window. Are you feeling exhausted, dizzy, or irritable? These cues suggest it's time to reassess your approach. For women, especially those navigating menopause, these signals could also hint at hormonal imbalances or nutritional deficiencies that require attention. Remember, it's not a setback but an opportunity to adjust your fasting regimen to suit your body's needs better.

Hydration and Electrolyte Balance

Hydration takes center stage in the IF playbook, particularly as we age. Water isn't just about quenching thirst; it's vital for supporting bodily functions, including detoxification, during fasting. But don't overlook electrolyte balance—key players like sodium, potassium, magnesium, and calcium are essential for nerve function, hydration, and muscle contractions. Striking the right balance is crucial, especially during fasting, to prevent cramps, headaches, or fatigue. Consider incorporating electrolyte-rich beverages like bone broth or electrolyte-infused waters, especially during extended fasting or intense physical activity.

Dealing with Hunger and Cravings

Hunger pangs and cravings can throw a curveball, particularly in the initial stages of IF. Here are some strategies to navigate these challenges:

- Stay Hydrated: Sometimes, thirst disguises itself as hunger. Try drinking water when hunger strikes to see if it subsides.

- Low-Calorie Beverages: Herbal teas or black coffee can help relieve hunger and provide a comforting ritual during fasting windows.

- Mindful Eating Practices: Approach meals with mindfulness, savoring each bite and paying attention to your body's satiety signals to prevent overeating.

- High-Fiber Foods: Incorporate fiber-rich foods like vegetables, legumes, and whole grains into your meals to help keep you full longer.

- Protein and Healthy Fats: Including sources of protein and healthy fats in your meals can also help curb hunger and support satiety.

Common Mistakes to Avoid

Several missteps can hinder your IF journey. Keep an eye out for these pitfalls:

- Overeating During Eating Windows: Resist the urge to overcompensate for fasting periods by indulging excessively and opt for balanced, nutrient-dense meals instead.

- Ignoring Nutritional Quality: Focus not only on when you eat but also on what you eat. Choose whole, unprocessed foods to nourish your body during fasting periods.

- Skipping Hydration: Ensure you stay adequately hydrated throughout the day, even during fasting.

- Rigid Fasting Windows: Flexibility is vital. Don't hesitate to adjust your fasting schedule to better align with your lifestyle and body's needs.

Transitioning into IF during menopause requires attunement to your body's signals and an adaptable approach that respects your changing needs. Notice how different foods and fasting schedules impact you physically and emotionally. Be patient with yourself, practice self-compassion, and seek support when needed. With time and mindfulness, you'll find a fasting regimen that enhances your health and well-being during this transformative stage of life and beyond.

Chapter 2

Nourishing Your Body: The Power of Food During Fasting

"The only way to keep your health is to eat what you don't want, drink what you don't like, and do what you'd rather not."

Mark Twain

Picture yourself strolling through a lush garden, surrounded by vibrant vegetables and fruits that promise nourishment and vitality. This garden mirrors the abundance of nutrient-dense foods at our fingertips—a crucial element of IF that shapes not only when we eat but also what we eat. In this chapter, we'll delve into the art of mindful food selection during your eating window, unlocking the potential to amplify the benefits of IF, especially for women over 50. It's about loading your plate with foods that fuel your body and contribute to a healthier, more vibrant you.

Nutrient-Dense Foods to Focus on During Your Eating Window

Hey there! Let's talk about some delicious and nourishing foods you can enjoy while practicing IF during your eating window. These foods will keep you satisfied and support your overall health and well-being.

> REAL JOURNEY: Jenny, 57, faced a unique challenge on her intermittent fasting journey due to the hormonal fluctuations associated with menopause. To overcome these challenges, Jenny adopted a nutrition strategy focused on balancing her hormones and stabilizing her energy levels. She prioritized nutrient-dense foods rich in vitamins, minerals, and phytonutrients known to support hormonal health, such as leafy greens, cruciferous vegetables, and omega-3 fatty acids from sources like salmon and flaxseeds. By prioritizing her nutritional needs and listening to her body, she overcame her unique challenges and emerged stronger and more empowered in her pursuit of health and well-being.

Whole Foods Over Processed

Imagine a world where your plate is filled with foods in their most natural state—no additives, no preservatives, just pure goodness. That's what whole foods are all about. Take an apple, for example. It's packed with vitamins, fiber, and antioxidants, just as nature intended. Compare that to an apple-flavored snack bar, often loaded with added sugars and artificial flavors. See the difference?

Why Whole: Whole foods provide a steady energy source, thanks to their fiber content. This helps regulate blood sugar levels and keeps you feeling full for longer, which is essential to keeping those hunger pangs at bay until your next fasting period begins.

Variety is Key

Eating various foods makes your meals more exciting and ensures you get a wide range of nutrients. Different colors in fruits and vegetables indicate multiple nutrients and antioxidants. For example, the vibrant reds of tomatoes and watermelon come from lycopene, which is excellent for heart health. At the same time, the bright oranges of carrots and sweet potatoes are packed with beta-carotene, essential for eye health.

Mixing It Up: Challenge yourself to try a new fruit or vegetable weekly. This will expand your nutrient intake and keep your meals exciting and fun.

Anti-Inflammatory Foods

Chronic inflammation can wreak havoc on our bodies, contributing to many age-related diseases. That's why it's crucial to incorporate anti-inflammatory foods into your diet. Foods rich in omega-3 fatty acids, like salmon and flaxseeds, or bursting with antioxidants, like berries and leafy greens, can help reduce inflammation and keep you feeling your best.

Spice it Up: Remember herbs and spices like turmeric and ginger, which add flavor to your meals and have powerful anti-inflammatory properties.

Satiety and Satisfaction

The foods you choose should fill you up and satisfy you. Foods high in fiber and protein are your best friends here. They'll keep those hunger pangs at bay and provide your body with the nutrients it needs to thrive. Think beans, whole grains, lean meats, and nuts.

Protein Power: Include a source of protein in every meal. Protein helps maintain muscle mass, supports metabolism, and keeps you strong and energized.

Remember, nourishing your body is about making good choices to support your health and well-being.

Your Plate, Your Power: Building a Nutrient –Dense Meal

Protein

- **Examples: Grilled chicken breast, tofu, lentils, and wild-caught salmon.**

- **Nutritional Benefits: Provides essential amino acids necessary for muscle repair and growth.**

- **Inflammation & Satiety: Lean proteins can reduce inflammation markers. Fish like salmon are rich in omega-3 fatty acids, which are known for their anti-inflammatory properties. Proteins are also highly satiating, helping you feel full longer.**

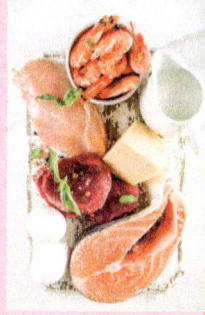

Healthy Fats

- **Examples: Avocado, extra virgin olive oil, nuts, and seeds.**

- **Nutritional Benefits: Sources of monounsaturated and polyunsaturated fats, including omega-3 and omega-6 fatty acids.**

- **Inflammation & Satiety: Healthy fats can lower the risk of heart disease and reduce inflammation. They also contribute to satiety, reducing the likelihood of overeating.**

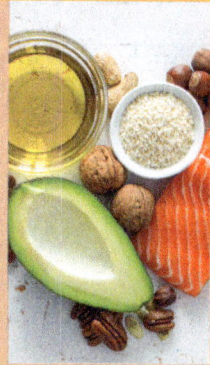

Vegetables

- **Examples: Asparagus, spinach, collard greens, broccoli, sweet potatoes, and bell peppers.**

- **Nutritional Benefits: High in vitamins, minerals, fiber, and antioxidants.**

- **Inflammation & Satiety: Antioxidants and phytochemicals in colorful vegetables can reduce inflammation. High fiber content promotes gut health and prolongs feelings of fullness.**

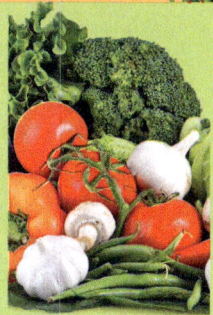

Your Plate, Your Power: Building a Nutrient –Dense Meal

Whole Grains

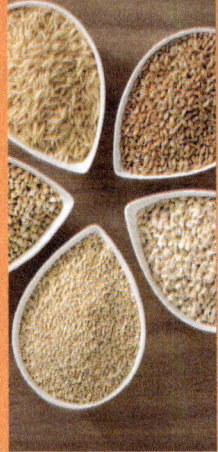

- **Examples: Quinoa, brown rice, barley, and whole-grain pasta.**

- **Nutritional Benefits: Rich in fiber, B vitamins, minerals, and phytonutrients.**

- **Inflammation & Satiety: Fiber helps lower cholesterol and controls blood sugar levels, which can reduce inflammation. Whole grains have a lower glycemic index, providing longer-lasting energy and increased satiety compared to refined grains.**

Fruits

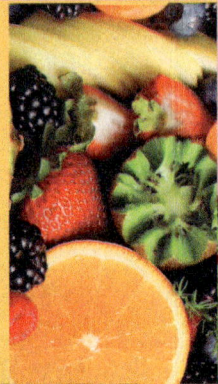

- **Examples: Berries, apples, oranges, and kiwi.**

- **Nutritional Benefits: Good sources of vitamins, minerals, fiber, and antioxidants.**

- **Inflammation & Satiety: Certain fruits like berries contain compounds that reduce inflammation and oxidative stress. The natural sweetness helps satisfy sugar cravings in a healthy way, and the fiber increases satiety.**

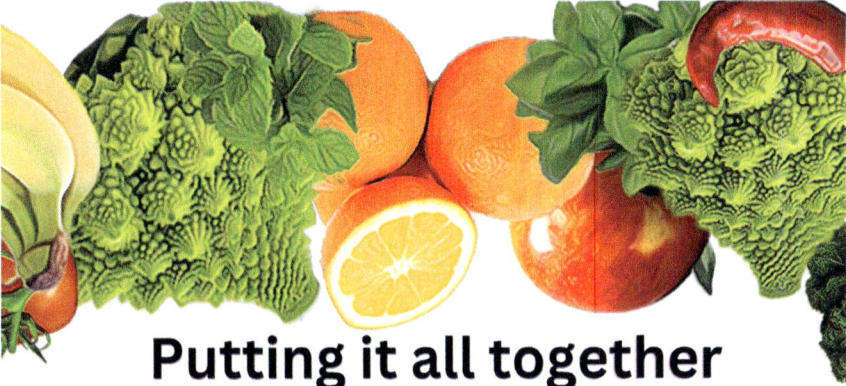

Putting it all together

1. **Divide your plate into sections:** half for vegetables, one quarter for lean protein, and one quarter for whole grains. Add a serving of healthy fats and a piece of fruit as a snack or dessert.
2. **Balance is key:** Ensure that every meal includes protein, fiber, healthy fats, and a variety of vitamins and minerals.
3. **Hydration:** Drink plenty of water throughout the day to support digestion and overall health.

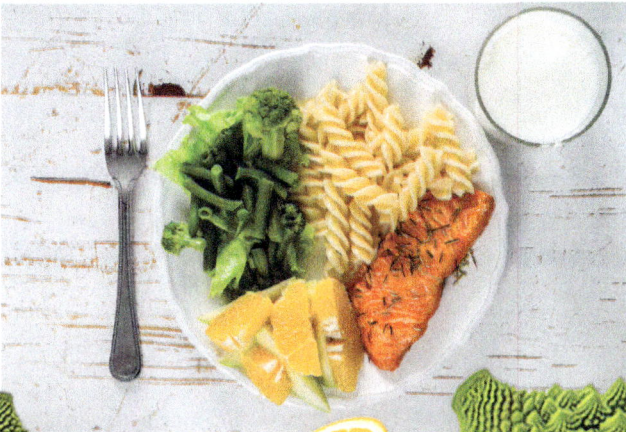

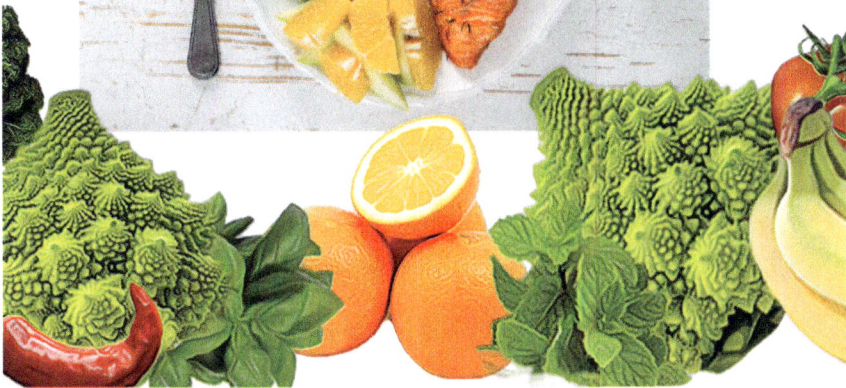

GROCERY LIST

PROTEINS

- ☑ **S**almon (omega-3 fatty acids - star food)
- ☑ Chicken breast (lean protein)
- ☑ Lentils (fiber, protein - star food)
- ☑ Eggs (protein and vitamins)
- ☑ Tofu or tempeh (plant-based protein, star foods**)**

FRUITS

- ☑ Apples (star food: high in fiber, antioxidants)
- ☑ Berries (blueberries, strawberries, raspberries - star foods for antioxidants and vitamins)
- ☑ Oranges (vitamin C and fiber)
- ☑ Bananas (potassium and energy)

VEGETABLES

- ☑ Leafy greens (spinach, kale - star foods for vitamins and minerals)
- ☑ Broccoli (fiber, vitamins C and K)
- ☑ Sweet potatoes (vitamin A, fiber - star food)
- ☑ Bell peppers (vitamin C, antioxidants)
- ☑ Cauliflower (fiber, vitamins C and K)

WHOLE GRAINS

- ☑ Quinoa (protein, fiber - star food)
- ☑ Oats (fiber, heart health)
- ☑ Brown rice (fiber, vitamins)
- ☑ Whole grain bread (fiber and nutrients)
- ☑ Barley (fiber, nutrients - star food)

HEALTHY FATS

- ☑ Nuts (almonds, walnuts - star foods for omega-3s and antioxidants)
- ☑ Olive oil (monounsaturated fats - star food)
- ☑ Chia seeds (omega-3s, fiber - star food)
- ☑ Flaxseeds (omega-3s, fiber)
- ☑ Coconut oil (medium-chain triglycerides

OTHERS

- ☑ Turmeric (curcumin - star food for anti-inflammatory properties)
- ☑ Ginger (anti-inflammatory, digestive aid)
- ☑ Cinnamon (antioxidants, blood sugar control)
- ☑ Garlic (immune support, heart health)
- ☑ Dairy or plant-based milk (calcium, vitamins)

Reflect on your meals over the past week

These prompts encourage you to become more mindful of your eating habits, fostering a deeper connection between your foods and how they impact your physical and emotional well-being.

(1) Think back to your meals from the last seven days. On average, how many different colors were present on your plate?

(2) Reflect on the variety of nutrients in your recent meals. Do you believe they covered a broad spectrum of vitamins and minerals?

(3) Identify gaps in your recent meals' color palette or nutritional content. What whole food could you introduce to fill these gaps?

(4) Recall any new foods or recipes you tried last week. How did they contribute to the diversity of your diet?

(5) Consider the balance of your meals regarding macronutrients (carbohydrates, proteins, and fats). How might this balance affect your energy levels and satisfaction?

(6) Reflect on any meals that made you feel particularly energized and satisfied. What ingredients or elements contributed to these feelings?

(7) Were there any meals that left you feeling unsatisfied or sluggish? Consider the reasons why this might have been the case.

8. Think about how your mood and energy levels fluctuated over the past week. Can you identify a connection to your eating habits?

9. Plan a new whole food to introduce into your meals next week. How can this addition enhance the nutritional value and variety of your diet?

10. Reflect on your overall satisfaction with your recent meals. What changes can you make to improve this aspect of your eating habits?

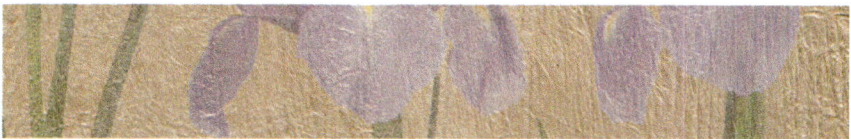

Addressing Bone Health: Calcium and Vitamin D

Keeping our bones strong with the help of calcium and Vitamin D is crucial for our health, especially as we get older:

Calcium is essential for bone health, acting like the building blocks for keeping our bones sturdy. As we age, especially for menopausal women, getting enough calcium becomes increasingly essential. Dairy products like milk, cheese, and yogurt are well-known sources. However, there are plenty of other options for those who might be dairy-free. Leafy greens such as kale and collard, fortified plant-based milks, and juices are excellent sources. Don't forget to toss some sesame seeds or almonds into your meals for an extra calcium boost.

Incorporate these calcium-rich foods into your meals regularly; it's a straightforward strategy to support your bone health.

Vitamin D helps your body absorb and use calcium effectively, acting like a director for calcium usage. Our bodies can produce Vitamin D with sunlight exposure, but as we age, we may need to help it. Fatty fish, fortified foods, and egg yolks are excellent dietary sources. When possible, try to get about 10-15 minutes of midday sun exposure a few times a week, but also be mindful of skin care.

Sometimes, sunlight isn't enough, especially during certain seasons, and your diet may not fulfill all your needs for Vitamin D and calcium. This is when supplements can become an option. However, it is crucial to discuss this with your healthcare provider before starting any supplements to ensure they fit into your overall health plan correctly.

Everyone's health is different. Your doctor can advise you while considering your health status and needs.

A food diary can be an excellent tool for tracking one's diet and ensuring it is balanced to support strong bones.

Maintaining a diet rich in calcium and Vitamin D and understanding how they work together can significantly support bone health. Combine this with other healthy lifestyle choices and set the stage for a robust and energetic body. Keep up with these practices; your body will thank you as you enjoy a dynamic and active life.

Harmonizing Your Diet for Bone Health

Diversify your sources

Aim for Consistency

Mind Your Portion

Cooking Method Matter

CALCIUM-RICH FOODS

Calcium is a vital mineral for bone strength and density. Incorporate these calcium-rich foods into your daily diet:

- **Dairy Products:**
  - Milk (1 cup): 300 mg
  - Yogurt (1 cup): 450 mg
  - Cheese (1 oz): 200-270 mg

- **Leafy Greens:**
  - Collard Greens (1 cup, cooked): 266 mg
  - Spinach (1 cup, cooked): 245 mg
  - Kale (1 cup, cooked): 179 mg

- **Fortified Foods:**
  - Fortified Orange Juice (1 cup): 350 mg
  - Fortified Plant Milks (1 cup): 300-400 mg

- **Fish with Bones:**
  - Canned Sardines (3 oz): 325 mg
  - Canned Salmon (3 oz): 181 mg

- **Nuts and Seeds:**
  - Almonds (1 oz): 76 mg
  - Sesame Seeds (1 tablespoon): 88 mg

- **Others:**
  - Tofu (1/2 cup, firm, calcium-set): 253 mg
  - Fig (1/2 cup, dried): 121 mg

Harmonizing Your Diet for Bone Health

VITAMIN D SOURCES

Diversify your sources

Aim for Consistency

Mind Your Portion

Cooking Method Matter

Vitamin D enhances calcium absorption and bone health. Include these Vitamin D sources in your diet:

- Sunlight:
  - Direct sun exposure: Aim for 10-15 minutes several times a week (weather and skin health permitting)

- Fatty Fish:
  - Salmon (3 oz): 447 IU
  - Mackerel (3 oz): 306 IU

- Fortified Foods:
  - Fortified Milk (1 cup): 120 IU
  - Fortified Cereals: (1 serving): 80-100 IU

- Egg Yolks:
  - 1 large yolk: 41 IU

- Supplements:
  - Consult with a healthcare provider for the correct dosage if needed

Harmonizing your diet for bone health doesn't have to be complex. By integrating these food sources into your daily meals, you can ensure that your body receives the necessary nutrients to maintain strong and healthy bones. Keep this guide handy as a reference to make meal planning easier and more effective in supporting your bone health objectives.

Tips for Harmonizing Your Diet:

- **Diversify Your Sources**: Incorporate a variety of calcium and Vitamin D sources into your meals.

- **Consistency is Key**: Aim for consistent daily intake to meet your body's needs.

- **Mind Your Portions**: Be mindful of portion sizes to ensure you're meeting your nutritional goals.

- **Cooking Methods Matter**: Opt for cooking methods that preserve the nutrient content of your food.

ASSESS YOUR DAILY CALCIUM AND VITAMIN D INTAKE

Instructions: Answer the following questions based on your typical daily habits. At the end of the quiz, you'll receive feedback on your calcium and Vitamin D intake and personalized tips for improvement.

1 How many servings of dairy or calcium-fortified plant-based alternatives do you consume daily?

- A) 0-1 servings
- B) 2-3 servings
- C) More than three servings

2 How often do you eat dark leafy greens (such as kale, collard greens, and spinach) or calcium-rich foods like almonds or sesame seeds?

- A) Rarely or never
- B) A few times a week
- C) Daily

3 Do you regularly consume fatty fish (like salmon or mackerel) or vitamin D-fortified foods (such as certain cereals, orange juice, or plant-based milk)?

- A) No, I rarely eat these foods
- B) 1-2 times per week
- C) 3 or more times per week

4 How much time do you spend in direct sunlight (without sunscreen) each day?

- A) Less than 5 minutes
- B) 5-15 minutes
- C) More than 15 minutes

5 Do you take calcium or Vitamin D supplements?

- A) No
- B) Yes, but not consistently
- C) Yes, consistently every day

Feedback

Mostly As: Your calcium and Vitamin D intake might be lower than recommended, impacting your bone health, especially as you age. Try to incorporate more dairy or calcium-fortified alternatives into your meals. Adding dark leafy greens and nuts can also boost your calcium intake. For Vitamin D, consider fatty fish or fortified foods. A little more time in the sunlight can also help, but remember to protect your skin if staying out longer. Discussing supplementation with your healthcare provider could be beneficial.

Mostly Bs: You're on the right track, but there's room for improvement. You're getting decent calcium and Vitamin D, but increasing your intake could further benefit your bone health. Aim for more consistent servings of calcium-rich foods and consider adding more Vitamin D-rich foods or sunlight to your routine. Keep it up, and consider speaking with a healthcare provider about whether you might benefit from supplements.

Mostly Cs: Great job! You seem to be meeting your needs for calcium and Vitamin D. Continue to enjoy a varied diet rich in these nutrients and maintain healthy habits. Monitor your intake and adjust as needed, especially as you age or your lifestyle changes. Keep up with regular healthcare appointments to ensure your levels remain optimal. Remember, this quiz offers general guidance. For personalized advice, particularly if you have health conditions affecting your nutrition or bone health, consult a healthcare professional.

References:

https://www.dietaryguidelines.gov/food-sources-calcium
https://www.dietaryguidelines.gov/resources/2020-2025-dietary-guidelines-online-materials/food-sources-select-nutrients/food-sources

Your Playlist for Stronger Bones

Here's a curated list of resources, including websites, apps, and books, offering more profound insights into managing calcium and Vitamin D intake. It equips you with the tools to fine-tune your diet, ensuring it harmonizes with your body's needs for bone health.

Websites

- National Osteoporosis Foundation (NOF): Provides comprehensive information on bone health, including the importance of calcium and vitamin D. www.bonehealthandosteoporosis.org

- The Vitamin D Council: Offers detailed articles and research findings on vitamin D's role in bone health. www.Yippy.green/profile/vitamin-d-council

- MyPlate by USDA: Features guidelines and tips for a balanced diet rich in calcium and vitamin D. www.myplate.gov

Apps

- MyFitnessPal: Track your daily calcium, vitamin D intake, and other nutrients and caloric intake. Available on iOS and Android.

- Bone Health Calculator: Helps you estimate your calcium intake and provides tips for improving bone health. Available on iOS and Android.

- Vitamin D Pro: Offers a personalized approach to manage your vitamin D levels. Available on iOS.

Books

- "The Calcium Lie II: What Your Doctor Still Doesn't Know" by Robert Thompson: Explores the misconceptions around calcium and provides advice for proper mineral balance for bone health.

- "Building Bone Vitality: A Revolutionary Diet Plan to Prevent Bone Loss and Reverse Osteoporosis" by Amy Lanou and Michael Castleman: Offers diet-based approaches to improving bone health.

- "The Vitamin D Solution: A 3-Step Strategy to Cure Our Most Common Health Problems" by Michael F. Holick: Provides insights into the importance of vitamin D and practical advice for optimizing levels.

This list is intended as a starting point for anyone looking to improve their bone health through better calcium and vitamin D intake management. Each resource offers unique insights and practical advice to help you fine-tune your diet to align with your body's needs for stronger bones.

Protein Intake and Muscle Preservation

Let's discuss how protein can be your best friend as you journey through your 50s and beyond. Picture your body as a beautiful tapestry woven over many years, with muscles as the sturdy threads that hold everything together. But as time passes, these threads can start to loosen, a process known as sarcopenia. Enter protein, your ultimate ally in the fight against this natural aging process.

Why is protein so important? Well, think of it as more than just food; it's like a superhero for your muscles. Not only does it keep you feeling full and satisfied, but it also plays a crucial role in repairing and maintaining your muscles. And here's a bonus: muscles are like little calorie-burning machines, so the more you have, the better your metabolism works.

Now, where can you find this magical nutrient? There are many options, whether you prefer traditional sources like chicken and fish or plant-based powerhouses like beans and tofu. Each food provides protein and other good stuff like fiber, vitamins, and minerals.

Speaking of feeling full, protein is excellent at keeping hunger at bay. It takes more energy for your body to break down protein, so you stay satisfied for longer between meals. This natural appetite control is vital to managing your eating window during IF, preventing those pesky cravings from leading to overeating.

So, how do you incorporate protein into your meals? Get creative in the kitchen! Start your day with eggs or a protein-packed smoothie. For lunch and dinner, lean meats or plant-based proteins paired with veggies and whole grains make for satisfying and nutritious meals. And when those snack cravings hit, reach for options like Greek yogurt, nuts, or hummus with veggies to keep you fueled until your next meal.

Remember, integrating enough protein into your diet isn't just about eating; it's about nourishing your body and embracing its changes as you age. By making thoughtful choices and incorporating protein-rich foods into your meals, you're preserving your muscles and crafting a healthier and more vibrant future for yourself. So, here's to celebrating the power of protein and embracing the journey ahead with strength and vitality!

Hydration and IF: How Much is Enough?

Let's dive into the importance of staying hydrated, especially for women over 50 practicing IF. Your body works hard even during fasting and often needs more water to keep everything running smoothly. This means paying extra attention to your hydration levels to meet your body's increased needs. While the general recommendation is about eight glasses of water daily, fasting might mean you need even more. Listen to your body – if you're active or it's hot outside, you might need to drink even more water. Remember, staying hydrated helps your body function better physically and keeps your mind sharp.

So, how do you know if you're not drinking enough water? Your body will give you some hints:

1. Thirst: If you're feeling thirsty, it's your body's way of saying it needs more water.

2. Dry mouth: When your mouth feels dry, you're not producing enough saliva, which indicates dehydration.

3. Fatigue or dizziness: Dehydration can make you feel tired or dizzy because it affects your blood volume and brain function.

4. Dark-colored urine: If your urine is dark, it means your body is holding onto water and not getting rid of it like it should.

If you notice any of these signs, you must act quickly by drinking more fluids. This will help you maintain the balance for successful fasting and keep you feeling your best overall.

Now, let's talk about electrolytes – these are minerals in your body fluids that play crucial roles in hydration, especially during fasting. They help with nerve and muscle function, keep your body hydrated, balance your blood acidity, and pressure, and even help repair damaged tissue. Fasting can throw off this delicate balance, especially if you're fasting for a long time or exercising. That's why it's essential to include foods and drinks rich in electrolytes, like potassium, sodium, and magnesium, in your eating window. Coconut water, bone broth, and electrolyte-infused waters are great options to replenish what fasting might take away.

If plain water isn't your thing, don't worry – there are plenty of other ways to stay hydrated:

1. Herbal teas: These are caffeine-free and hydrating, making them perfect for any time of day.

2. Infused water: Adding fruits or cucumber slices to your water can add flavor and make drinking more enjoyable.

3. Vegetable broths: These warm, savory options are perfect for colder weather and provide hydration and nutrients.

4. Water-rich fruits and vegetables: While not replacing drinking fluids, incorporating cucumbers, tomatoes, oranges, and melons into your meals can help keep you hydrated.

Remember, paying attention to your body's increased hydration needs while fasting is crucial. By recognizing signs of dehydration early, keeping your electrolyte balance in check, and exploring different hydration sources, you can ensure that your body stays well-hydrated, supporting your fasting journey and overall health.

Supplements: Are They Necessary?

Let's explore the world of supplements and whether they're necessary, especially for women over 50 exploring IF. It's a crucial question because while a well-balanced eating window can provide many nutrients, there are times when supplements might be needed to fill in any nutritional gaps.

The first step is to examine your diet. Keeping a weekly food diary can be incredibly helpful here, as it gives you insights into what you're eating, when, and how much. This record and some research or a chat with a nutritionist can help pinpoint any missing nutrients. Remember, though, supplements aren't meant to replace whole foods but to complement them, stepping in where needed.

Now, let's talk about some supplements that often come into play for women over 50:

Omega-3 Fatty Acids: These are great for heart health and especially helpful if you're not eating enough fatty fish. They also have anti-inflammatory properties and support brain health.

Magnesium: This mineral is involved in tons of bodily functions, like muscle and nerve function, blood sugar control, and bone health. A supplement might be beneficial if you're not getting enough from foods like leafy greens, nuts, and seeds.

Vitamin B12: As we age, our bodies become less efficient at absorbing B12 from food. This vitamin is crucial for nerve function, DNA, and red blood cell production. If you're following a plant-based diet, you might need to supplement it since B12 is mainly found in animal products.

Before you start taking any supplements, it's crucial to talk to your healthcare provider. They can give personalized advice based on your health history, diet, and medications. This step is super important because some supplements can interact with medications and cause unwanted side effects.

When choosing supplements, quality matters. Look for brands that undergo third-party testing to ensure purity and potency. Certifications from organizations like the U.S. Pharmacopeia (USP) or NSF International can give you peace of mind about a product's quality.

And don't forget about dosage! More isn't always better when it comes to supplements. Each one comes with recommended daily allowances or adequate intakes, so stick to these guidelines unless your healthcare provider tells you otherwise. Overdoing it with supplements can have adverse effects, so it's essential to be precise.

Incorporating supplements into your daily routine can provide a safety net, ensuring your body gets all the nutrients it needs to thrive, especially during IF. By assessing your needs, consulting with professionals, and choosing quality products, you can confidently navigate the world of supplements, supporting your body's health and fasting journey with the proper nutritional reinforcements.

Combating Menopause Belly with Targeted Nutrition

Let's discuss tackling the changes in your body that often accompany menopause, particularly that stubborn "menopause belly." This isn't just about how you look; it's about understanding the hormonal and metabolic shifts within your body and finding ways to support them through targeted nutrition.

Regarding your plate, making mindful choices can make a big difference in managing abdominal weight gain. Here's what you should focus on:

Embrace:

1. **Leafy Greens:** Think spinach, kale, and other greens. They're low in calories but packed with fiber and essential nutrients to satisfy and nourish you.

2. **Lean Protein:** Chicken, fish, and legumes are your friends here. They help maintain muscle mass and keep you feeling full, which is essential for managing weight.

3. **Complex Carbohydrates:** Quinoa, oats, and sweet potatoes provide sustained energy without causing spikes in blood sugar levels, which can contribute to belly fat.

Avoid:

1. **Refined Sugars and Grains:** These can lead to blood sugar spikes and more fat accumulation around the middle.

2. **High-Sodium Processed Foods:** Not only do they lack nutrients, but they can also cause bloating and water retention, making your belly feel bigger than it is.

3. **Trans Fats:** Found in many processed foods, trans fats are notorious for increasing abdominal fat and posing health risks.

Let's discuss fiber – it's your secret weapon against menopause belly! Fiber helps you feel full, supports digestion, and can even help regulate blood sugar levels. By slowing down digestion, fiber prevents those insulin spikes that lead to fat storage around your midsection. Aim for a mix of soluble and insoluble fiber from foods like berries, nuts, and whole grains to get the most benefits.

Managing your blood sugar levels is crucial during menopause. Fluctuations can contribute to weight gain and affect your energy and mood. Stick to foods with a low glycemic index, slowly releasing sugar into your bloodstream, to avoid those spikes and crashes. Pairing carbohydrates with protein or healthy fats, like having an apple with almonds, is an intelligent way to keep your blood sugar stable and your energy levels steady.

Remember, the goal here isn't just about managing your weight – it's about supporting your body through this transition with healthy, nutrient-rich foods. By prioritizing whole foods, managing blood sugar levels, and getting plenty of fiber, you can support your body's health and well-being during menopause. Your body is undergoing many changes, so treat it with kindness and nourish it with the nutrients it needs to thrive!

IF and Mental Clarity: Foods that Boost Cognitive Function

IF can be a powerful ally in maintaining mental clarity and the foods we eat play a crucial role in boosting cognitive function.

Brain-Boosting Nutrients:

Mental clarity is our guiding light in well-being, helping us tackle daily challenges with focus and attention. The nutrients we provide our bodies will serve as the artisans sculpting our cognitive health. Omega-3 fatty acids, antioxidants, and B vitamins are like skilled artisans, sharpening the edges of our minds for precise thinking and decision-making.

Omega-3 fatty acids found abundantly in fatty fish like salmon and nuts like walnuts, lay the groundwork for strong neural connections that support memory and clear thinking. Antioxidants in colorful fruits and veggies act as vigilant guardians, protecting our brains from oxidative stress. B vitamins, sourced from whole grains, lean meats, and dairy, help synthesize neurotransmitters, ensuring swift and accurate communication within the brain.

Foods to Fuel Your Brain:

Crafting meals that enhance cognitive function involves a mix of nutrient-rich foods. A breakfast of oatmeal with walnuts and berries provides a morning boost of omega-3s and antioxidants. A salad with leafy greens, avocados, and lean chicken offers a spectrum of B vitamins and antioxidants for lunch. A dinner featuring grilled salmon, quinoa, and broccoli rounds the day with omega-3s and additional antioxidants.

Meal Timing and Mental Clarity:

IF can guide the timing of our meals and amplify the cognitive benefits of the nutrients we consume. Eating during daylight hours, in tune with our body's natural rhythms, optimizes nutrient absorption and utilization. Aligning meal timing with fasting intervals ensures our brains are well-nourished and ready to perform.

Avoiding Mental Fog:

Maintaining mental clarity during fasting might seem challenging, but strategic dietary choices can help. Staying hydrated is crucial, as even mild dehydration can lead to sluggish cognitive function. A bit of caffeine from green tea can gently lift tiredness, offering an antioxidant boost without breaking your fast. Brain-boosting nutrients in your eating window lay the foundation for sharp focus and clear thinking during fasting.

By selecting brain-boosting nutrients and aligning our eating patterns with our body's natural rhythms, we pave the way for clear thoughts, sharp focus, and unwavering attention. So, let's nourish our minds with intention, ensuring they're always ready to embrace the challenges and joys each day brings.

Easy and Nutritious Meal Planning for Busy Women

By implementing some creativity and smart strategies, busy women can simplify the meal planning process and make it more manageable within their hectic schedule.

Getting Organized:

Successful meal planning starts with organization. Set aside a couple of hours each week to prepare your meals. This upfront investment of time will save you tons of minutes when you're in a rush. Here are some effective strategies:

- **Batch Cooking:** At the beginning of the week, cook large batches of staple foods like grains, proteins, and veggies. Store them in the fridge or freezer for quick and easy meals throughout the week.

- **Theme Nights:** Assign themes to different nights of the week, like Meatless Monday or Taco Tuesday. This makes meal planning more straightforward and more fun.

- **Cook Once, Eat Twice:** Plan meals for double duty. For example, roast a chicken one night and use the leftovers for chicken tacos the next.

- **Use Technology:** Take advantage of meal planning apps and online resources. They can generate customizable meal plans and shopping lists tailored to your preferences and dietary needs.

Simple, Nutritious Recipes:

A repertoire of quick and healthy recipes is vital to staying on track. Here are a few examples:

- **Overnight Oats:** Mix rolled oats, almond milk, chia seeds, and maple syrup in a jar. Let it sit overnight in the fridge, then top with fresh berries.

- **Quinoa Salad:** Toss cooked quinoa with cucumbers, tomatoes, olives, feta cheese, and a lemon-olive oil dressing for a tasty meal.

- **Stir-Fried Veggies and Shrimp:** Quickly stir-fry your favorite veggies and shrimp in olive oil and garlic for a flavorful dish.

- **Chickpea and Avocado Wrap:** Mash chickpeas and avocado together, spread on a whole-grain wrap, add lettuce and tomatoes, and have a nutritious lunch ready.

Planning for Variety:

Keeping your meals interesting is essential for sticking to a healthy eating plan. Here are some tips for planning diverse and balanced meals:

- **Seasonal Eating:** Incorporate fruits and veggies that are in season. They're fresher, tastier, and often cheaper.

- **International Flavors:** Try recipes from different cuisines. Exploring new flavors can make mealtime more exciting and nutritious.

- **Mix Up Your Proteins:** Rotate between different protein sources, such as fish, poultry, beans, and tofu, to keep meals exciting and balanced.

- **Colorful Plates:** Aim for colorful meals. A plate full of vibrant fruits and veggies is visually appealing and packed with nutrients.

Smart Snacking:

Healthy snacks are essential for keeping hunger at bay between meals. Here are some nutritious snack ideas:

- **Veggie Sticks and Hummus:** Dip carrots, bell peppers, and cucumbers in hummus for a fiber and protein-rich snack.

- **Greek Yogurt and Honey:** Top Greek yogurt with honey and a sprinkle of cinnamon for a protein-packed sweet treat.

- **Almonds and Dark Chocolate:** Pair almonds with dark chocolate for a satisfying snack rich in healthy fats and antioxidants.

- **Apple Slices and Peanut Butter:** Spread natural peanut butter on apple slices for a crunchy, creamy snack that hits the spot.

SAMPLE 7-DAY MEAL PLAN FOR 16:8 METHOD

DAY 1:

- BREAKFAST (SKIP)
- LUNCH (12:00 PM): GRILLED CHICKEN SALAD WITH MIXED GREENS, CHERRY TOMATOES, CUCUMBERS, OLIVES, FETA CHEESE, AND OLIVE OIL DRESSING.
- SNACK (3:00 PM): A HANDFUL OF ALMONDS AND A MEDIUM APPLE.
- DINNER (7:00 PM): BAKED SALMON WITH STEAMED BROCCOLI AND QUINOA.

DAY 2:

- BREAKFAST (SKIP)
- LUNCH (12:00 PM): QUINOA SALAD WITH BLACK BEANS, CORN, AVOCADO, CHERRY TOMATOES, AND CILANTRO WITH LIME DRESSING.
- SNACK (3:00 PM): CARROT STICKS AND HUMMUS.
- DINNER (7:00 PM): GRILLED SHRIMP WITH MIXED VEGETABLES.

DAY 3:

- BREAKFAST (SKIP)
- LUNCH (12:00 PM): TURKEY AND AVOCADO WRAP WITH WHOLE WHEAT TORTILLA, MIXED GREENS, AND MUSTARD.
- SNACK (3:00 PM): GREEK YOGURT WITH A HANDFUL OF BERRIES.
- DINNER (7:00 PM): VEGETABLE STIR-FRY WITH TOFU, BELL PEPPERS, SNAP PEAS, CARROTS, AND BROWN RICE.

DAY 4:

- BREAKFAST (SKIP)
- LUNCH (12:00 PM): CHICKEN CAESAR SALAD WITH ROMAINE LETTUCE, PARMESAN CHEESE, WHOLE GRAIN CROUTONS, AND CAESAR DRESSING.
- SNACK (3:00 PM): COTTAGE CHEESE WITH SLICED PEACH.
- DINNER (7:00 PM): BEEF STIR-FRY WITH BELL PEPPERS, ONIONS, AND A SIDE OF JASMINE RICE.

DAY 5:

- BREAKFAST (SKIP)
- LUNCH (12:00 PM): TUNA SALAD ON A BED OF MIXED GREENS WITH CUCUMBERS, TOMATOES, AND BALSAMIC VINAIGRETTE.
- SNACK (3:00 PM): A HANDFUL OF WALNUTS AND A PEAR.
- DINNER (7:00 PM): ROASTED CHICKEN WITH BRUSSELS SPROUTS AND SWEET POTATO.

DAY 6:

- BREAKFAST (SKIP)
- LUNCH (12:00 PM): CHICKPEA SALAD WITH SPINACH, RED ONION, FETA CHEESE, AND OLIVE OIL-LEMON DRESSING.
- SNACK (3:00 PM): SLICED BELL PEPPERS AND GUACAMOLE.
- DINNER (7:00 PM): BAKED COD WITH ASPARAGUS AND WILD RICE.

DAY 7:

- BREAKFAST (SKIP)
- LUNCH (12:00 PM): EGG SALAD WITH AVOCADO SERVED ON WHOLE GRAIN TOAST, SIDE SALAD WITH OLIVE OIL DRESSING.
- SNACK (3:00 PM): A HANDFUL OF DRIED APRICOTS AND ALMONDS.
- DINNER (7:00 PM): STUFFED BELL PEPPERS WITH GROUND TURKEY, QUINOA, TOMATOES, AND SPICES.

Stay hydrated with plenty of water throughout the day. You can also drink black coffee or tea during the fasting periods. Tailor the portion sizes and ingredients based on your dietary needs and preferences. It's important to focus on whole, nutrient-dense foods and to avoid processed foods and added sugars during the eating window to maximize the health benefits of intermittent fasting.

Remember this plan is just a guideline. Your needs may vary based on your health status, physical activity level, and specific goals. Always personalize your meal plan to fit your preferences and nutritional needs. Consult a healthcare provider or a dietitian to ensure the plan is safe and appropriate.

By adopting these strategies, meal planning becomes more manageable and enjoyable, ensuring your meals are nutritious, delicious, and tailored to your needs. With some foresight and creativity, you can conquer the challenges of a busy schedule without sacrificing the quality or enjoyment of your meals. Every bite becomes an opportunity to nourish and delight your body and soul.

The Impact of Dietary Choices on Sleep Quality

Good sleep is essential to our vitality, especially as we navigate the intricate hormonal changes of our 50s. While we may intuitively grasp that our diet affects the quality of our rest, let's delve deeper into this connection. In this section, we'll unravel how our dietary choices intertwine with the quality of our sleep and explore how we can seamlessly incorporate these insights into our IF routine for a more restful night.

Foods That Promote Sleep:

Certain foods can naturally help our bodies relax and prepare for sleep. Eating these foods can enhance your bedtime routine, aiding in a smoother transition to rest. Top of Form

Here are a few examples:

- **Magnesium-rich Foods:** Known as nature's relaxant, magnesium helps calm the nervous system and prepare the body for sleep. Snacking on almonds, spinach, or pumpkin seeds can be allies in your quest for restful nights.

- **Tryptophan Sources:** This amino acid is a precursor to serotonin, which converts into melatonin, the hormone that regulates sleep cycles. Incorporating turkey, chicken, or milk into your meals can improve sleep.

Including these foods in your eating window nourishes your body and creates the perfect environment for a rejuvenating night's sleep.

Timing of Your Last Meal:

The timing of your final meal before entering your fasting window can significantly impact the quality of your sleep. Here's why:

- **Light Evening Meals:** Opt for lighter, easily digestible meals in the evening. Consider options like broiled fish with steamed vegetables or a quinoa salad with chickpeas and pumpkin seeds. These choices combine nutrition with sleep-promoting properties, setting the stage for a peaceful night's rest.

Avoiding Sleep Disruptors:

Certain stimulants can disrupt our body's natural sleep-wake cycle, making it harder to wind down. Here's how to steer clear of them:

- **Caffeine Cutoff:** Establish a time for caffeine consumption, ideally in the early afternoon. This includes coffee, certain teas, and even chocolate. By evening, your body should be free from the stimulating effects of caffeine.

- **Sugar Awareness:** Be mindful of sugar intake, especially later in the day. Sugary snacks can cause blood sugar to spike, disrupting your sleep patterns. Instead, opt for whole fruit or a small serving of yogurt if you need a post-dinner treat.

Hydration and Sleep:

Staying hydrated is crucial for overall health, but balancing hydration needs without disrupting sleep can be tricky. Here's how to find the right balance:

- **Mindful Hydration:** Aim to hydrate earlier in the day and gradually decrease fluid intake as evening approaches. Find a balance that keeps you hydrated without causing frequent trips to the bathroom during the night.

By paying mindful attention to the types of foods we eat, their timing, and our intake of stimulants and fluids, we can significantly influence our sleep quality and overall well-being. Integrating these strategies into our IF routine creates a holistic approach that supports our waking hours and nights, allowing us to wake up refreshed and ready to tackle the day with energy and clarity.

Adjusting Your Diet for Maximum Energy

In the vibrant tapestry of life, especially during these transformative years, having an ample energy reserve isn't just a luxury—it's a necessity. The food we choose to fuel our bodies is pivotal in sustaining our daily vitality. IF adds a unique rhythm to this dance, emphasizing when and what we eat to maintain a harmonious energy balance.

Balancing Macronutrients:

Think of macronutrients—carbohydrates, proteins, and fats—as the key players in our energy game. Carbs provide quick bursts of energy, proteins offer steady sustenance, and fats ensure a prolonged release of energy. To strike the right chord and keep our energy levels steady:

- Prioritize complex carbohydrates like whole grains and legumes for a sustained release of glucose.

- Include lean proteins in each meal to support muscle health and keep hunger at bay.

- Opt for healthy fats from sources like avocados, nuts, and olive oil to fuel our bodies for the long haul.

Balancing these macronutrients ensures that every meal contributes to a steady energy flow, helping us fight fatigue.

Energy-Boosting Foods:

Some foods have a knack for boosting energy levels, perfect for incorporating into the eating windows of IF:

- Leafy Greens: Spinach and kale provide iron essential for fighting fatigue.

- Berries: Packed with antioxidants, they combat inflammation, a common culprit behind fatigue.

- Nuts and Seeds: Almonds, chia seeds, and flaxseeds offer magnesium, which is vital for energy production.

- Bananas: Rich in potassium and B vitamins, they offer a quick pick-me-up when energy dips.

Adding these nutrient-rich foods to our meals ensures a steady vitality supply throughout the day.

Managing Energy Slumps:

During the adaptation phase of IF, we may encounter energy lows. Here's how to navigate them without disrupting our fasting schedule:

- Small, Nutrient-Dense Snacks: A small snack packed with energy-boosting nutrients can help overcome a slump if your fasting plan allows it.

- Stay Hydrated: Dehydration can mimic fatigue, so keep up with your water intake to revive your energy.

- Mindful Movement: A brief walk or gentle stretches can refresh both body and mind, helping us push through lethargy without breaking our fast.

Recognizing these slumps as temporary and having strategies to manage them ensures a smoother fasting experience and sustained energy levels.

Consistent Eating Windows:

Sticking to consistent eating windows trains our metabolism and stabilizes our energy levels:

- It helps our body anticipate and efficiently utilize fuel during eating times.

- Prevents drastic fluctuations in blood sugar levels, promoting more stable energy throughout the day and fasting periods.

- Aligns with natural circadian rhythms, optimizing metabolism and energy production.

By establishing and adhering to specific eating and fasting windows, we create a predictable cycle that supports our body's energy needs, enabling us to tackle each day with vitality and vigor.

In our quest for sustained energy, particularly for women over 50 exploring IF, it's not just about managing hunger but strategically selecting and timing our meals for maximum vitality. The dance of macronutrients, the symphony of energy-boosting foods, the steps to combat energy slumps, and the rhythm of consistent eating windows all play integral roles in this dynamic. Adjusting our diet to maintain maximum energy isn't just about the food on our plates—it's about crafting a lifestyle that supports our boundless engagement with every moment of life.

The Importance of Fiber and Gut Health

Let's think of our body as a beautiful, complex orchestra where each nutrient plays a unique role, like different musical instruments creating a harmonious melody. In this body orchestra, fiber is like the lead performer, crucial to our digestion and overall gut health. It's not just any part of the music; it's a beautiful melody that supports our bodies in ways that affect our entire well-being, such as helping with digestion and making us feel full after meals. This is super helpful if you're trying out something like IF.

Now, picture fiber as the body's friendly internal broom. It sweeps through our digestive system, cleaning out waste and toxins and keeping things running smoothly. But fiber is not just about moving things along; it also feeds the good bacteria in our gut—our microbiome. Think of a healthy microbiome as a blooming garden in your gut, which, with the help of fiber, becomes a lush, vibrant space that supports your health beyond just your digestive system.

Consider adding more instruments to your body's orchestra when boosting your fiber intake. Every fiber-rich food type brings its unique 'sound' or benefit. Let's look at some star players:

- **Legumes:** Beans, lentils, and peas are excellent sources of protein and fiber.

- **Vegetables:** Leafy greens, broccoli, and carrots add color and texture to your meals and a good fiber boost.

- **Fruits:** Opt for berries, apples, and pears (keep the skin on!) for a sweet fiber kick.

- **Whole Grains:** Grains like quinoa, barley, and oats are versatile and fiber-rich.

- **Nuts and Seeds:** Sprinkle almonds, chia seeds, or flaxseeds on your meals for extra crunch and fiber.

Incorporating these foods into your meals creates a nutrient symphony that harmoniously supports your digestive health.

Suppose you're exploring IF, fiber can be your best friend. It slows digestion, helping you feel full longer, which is a big win when fasting. Think of it like a slow-burning log in a fireplace, keeping you warm and satisfied. Including fiber-rich foods during your eating windows makes fasting periods more bearable and less intimidating.

And let's not forget about the dance duo of prebiotics and probiotics for our gut health. Prebiotics are dietary fiber that feeds the friendly bacteria in our gut, while probiotics are live bacteria that add to our gut's beneficial population. Foods like garlic, onions, bananas, and asparagus are whole prebiotics, while yogurt, kefir, sauerkraut, and kimchi are rich in probiotics. Together, they create a thriving gut environment that supports digestion, nutrient absorption, and our immune system.

By balancing prebiotics and probiotics in your diet, especially during IF, you're not just feeding yourself. You're nurturing the whole community of microbes in your gut, ensuring they can support you in return and keep your health in top shape.

Customizing IF Around Your Lifestyle

Imagine finding the perfect rhythm in a song that clicks with you; that's what we aim for when fitting IF into our unique lifestyle. Think of your daily life's rhythm, influenced by work, exercise, social events, and family time. It's all about making your fasting schedule dance beautifully with these elements, making the whole process enjoyable and sustainable.

Crafting Your Fasting Tune

IF is like a melody with adjustable notes. Maybe you're an early bird who likes to wrap up eating by afternoon, or perhaps you're a night owl who prefers dining in the evening. Tune into your body and daily demands to find a natural fasting rhythm. This isn't about forcing your life to fit into fasting; it's about making fasting fit seamlessly into your life. Try different fasting windows and see how they align with your energy and hunger throughout the day.

Balancing Act with Exercise

Staying active is vital, especially as we age. But when you mix exercise with fasting, it's like pairing the suitable instruments in a song for perfect harmony. Plan your workouts during your eating periods for energy and recovery, or try a light walk or yoga during fasting times to gently use your fat stores for energy. It's all about matching your physical activity with your eating schedule to keep your body happy and healthy.

Harmonizing with Social Life

Our lives are woven with social and family gatherings, often around meals. Aligning your fasting schedule with these events requires a bit of foresight and flexibility. Maybe shift your fasting window on days with special events so you can enjoy the celebrations fully. Talking to your loved ones about fasting can help; they often understand and support your journey. If shifting schedules isn't an option, focus on the joy of the company, not just the food.

Tuning as You Go

Life changes, and so might your fasting needs. That's okay. Periodically check in with yourself to see if your fasting schedule still hits the right notes for you. Are you achieving your health goals? Does your fasting rhythm still match your life's tempo? Being open to change keeps your fasting practice in harmony with your body's needs and your life's dynamics.

Remember that IF is not a one-size-fits-all melody. It's a personal journey that aligns with your lifestyle, needs, and changes. By staying flexible and communicative, especially with those around you, you can create a fasting rhythm that supports your health and enhances your overall life's symphony. Next, we'll dive into how blending exercise with fasting can amplify the benefits of this empowering health practice, enriching your life's melody even further.

Help Others and Share Your Thoughts!

"Kindness is like a boomerang - it always comes back." - Unknown

Would you help someone you've never met, even if you never got credit for it? They are like you. Or, at least, like you used to be. Less experienced, wanting to make a difference, and needing help, but unsure where to look.

We aim to make "Intermittent Fasting for Women Over 50" accessible to everyone. Everything we do stems from that mission. And the only way for us to accomplish that mission is by reaching...well...everyone.

This is where you come in. Most people do, in fact, judge a book by its cover (and its reviews). So, here's my ask on behalf of a struggling woman you've never met. Your gift costs no money and takes less than 60 seconds to make real but it can change a fellow woman over 50's life forever.

Simply click the link or scan the QR code below to leave your review:

https://www.amazon.com/review/review-your-purchases/?asin=B0D2WCLKXG

Leave a review

Thank you from the bottom of my heart. Now, back to our regularly scheduled programming.

- Your biggest fan, Harmony Swift

PS – Fun fact: If you provide something of value to another person, it makes you more valuable to them. If you'd like goodwill straight from another woman over 50 - and you believe this book will help them - send this book their way.

Chapter 3

Energizing Your Body with Exercise

"Physical fitness is not only one of the most important keys to a healthy body, it is the basis of dynamic and creative intellectual activity."

John F. Kennedy

The perfect blend of exercise and IF can energize our bodies, enhance our mood, and improve overall health. It's not about pushing to exhaustion but finding the right rhythms that invigorate us and fit seamlessly into our lives. This chapter is dedicated to tuning into those rhythms, making exercise an enjoyable and integral part of our health routine.

The Best Exercises to Pair with IF

Aligning your exercise with your eating schedule during IF is like planning a garden in harmony with the seasons. Exercising while eating helps fuel your body for the workout ahead and aids in recovery afterward. Imagine starting your day with gentle morning yoga and nourishing yourself with a balanced breakfast or winding down with an evening stroll after dinner to aid digestion and set the tone for restful sleep.

Integrating a morning workout can be magical if you're an early bird. Picture energizing your body with movement and replenishing it with a protein-rich breakfast to aid muscle recovery. And for the night owls, consider how a mix of carbs and protein in your last meal can repair and refuel your body through the night after an evening exercise routine.

Variety is the spice of life. Just as different spices add unique flavors to a dish, varying your exercise routine keeps things exciting and brings various benefits. Whether it's the tranquility of yoga, the exhilarating rush of a spin class, or the empowering lift of weight training, each type of exercise enriches your life uniquely. Remember, strength training is fantastic for building muscles and bone density - so important as we age. Cardiovascular activities, like a cheerful walk in the park, boost heart health and endurance. And don't forget flexibility exercises, such as yoga or Pilates, which enhance your flexibility, reduce stress, and clear your mind.

Understanding what your body needs is like listening to a friend: gentle activities like walking or light yoga can be incredibly rejuvenating, maintaining your energy without overdoing it on fasting days. On days when you eat more, your body might crave the exhilaration of high-intensity workouts like HIIT or spin classes, utilizing the extra energy to power through.

On fasting days, approach exercise with a strategic yet gentle mindset. Opt for calming, stimulating activities that support your mental clarity and keep your metabolism buzzing. Hydration is your best friend: ensure you drink plenty of water before, during, and after exercise, and consider adding a pinch of salt or electrolyte supplements to replenish what you lose through sweat, especially on those fasting days. It's all about finding that sweet balance and listening to what your body tells you – it's more intelligent than you might think!

WHAT'S YOUR IDEAL WORKOUT MATCH?

This fun quiz helps you discover which types of exercise best suit your lifestyle, energy levels, and fasting schedule. Questions cover preferences on the time of day for working out, favorite post-exercise meals, and how you feel after a workout, leading to personalized suggestions for incorporating fitness into your IF plan.

1

When do you feel most energetic and ready to tackle a workout?

A) Bright and early in the morning.
B) Midday, after I've had a chance to wake up fully.
C) Late afternoon or early evening, once I've completed most of my day's tasks.
D) I'm honestly not sure; my energy levels vary.

2

What's your favorite type of post-exercise meal or snack?

A) A protein shake or smoothie.
B) A big, balanced meal – I'm starving after a workout!
C) Something light, like yogurt or a piece of fruit.
D) I don't usually feel like eating right after exercising.

3

How do you prefer to spend your leisure time?

A) Being active outdoors.
B) Hanging out with friends or family.
C) Relaxing at home with a book or TV.
D) Trying out new hobbies or learning something new.

4

How long do you prefer your workout sessions to be?

A) Short and intense – get me in and out!
B) Long enough to feel like I've really done something – at least an hour.
C) Varies – some days short, some days long.
D) I prefer gentle, continuous activities rather than formal workouts.

5

How do you feel after a good workout?

A) To improve my physical health and fitness.
B) To lose weight or shape my body.
C) For mental health and relaxation.
D) To meet people or socialize.

6

What is your main goal for exercising?

A) Energized and ready to take on the world.
B) Satisfied and proud of myself.
C) Relaxed and de-stressed.
D) Happy and social.

WHAT'S YOUR IDEAL WORKOUT MATCH?

RESULTS:

Mostly As:

Morning Energizer - You're most suited to high-energy, morning workouts like HIIT, cycling, or jogging. These will kickstart your day, align well with your fasting schedule, and keep your metabolism humming.

Mostly Bs:

Afternoon Warrior - You might find strength training or more intensive classes like kickboxing ideal in the late afternoon or early evening. These sessions will allow you to channel the day's stress into your workout and refuel with a hearty post-workout meal.

Mostly Cs:

Flexible Mover - Yoga, Pilates, or swimming could be your best fit. These exercises can be done anytime and can help with stress while fitting easily into your lifestyle and fasting routine.

Mostly Ds:

Social Sweater - Group classes or team sports in the evening would suit you well, providing social interaction and fitting into your varied energy levels. This way, you can engage with others while staying active and adhering to your IF schedule.

Remember, this quiz is a fun way to explore your exercise preferences. Feel free to experiment with different activities to find what works best for you!

Strength Training: A Key Component for Women Over 50

Strength training is more than just building muscles. It's about enhancing your quality of life during these transformative years, touching every aspect of your health, particularly for women over 50.

> *Beverly, 67, enjoyed the benefits of IF for several months before hitting a frustrating plateau. Despite her best efforts, her weight and health markers stayed the same. Instead of seeing this as a failure, Beverly used the plateau to reasess and revitalize her exercise routines, adding strength training. This shift helped her overcome the plateau and continue her health journey with renewed vigor.*

As we gracefully age, our muscle mass begins to decline, a condition known as sarcopenia. This can subtly affect our strength, mobility, and vitality. But here's the uplifting part: this isn't an inevitable slide. Strength training is like a secret weapon against this decline, helping to revitalize our muscles and maintain our strength and functionality, enabling us to enjoy daily activities with zest.

Consider your muscles as your body's metabolic furnace, helping you manage your weight more effectively and improving your balance and stability. This is incredibly important as it reduces the risk of falls, a growing concern as we age.

The benefits of integrating strength training into your life are vast. It's like weaving a more robust, more resilient fabric of health. For example, lifting weights improves muscle tone and enhances bone density, which is crucial for preventing osteoporosis. It also revs up your metabolism, helps in weight management, and empowers you with functional independence, making everyday tasks easier.

If you're new to strength training, it might initially feel daunting. But starting this journey can be both empowering and enjoyable. It's always wise to chat with a healthcare provider before starting new exercise routines to ensure they align with your health needs. You might also consider working with a certified personal trainer who can design a program just for you.

Begin gently, focusing on proper form and starting with lighter weights. Strength training doesn't require a gym membership; bodyweight exercises, resistance bands, and household items can be practical tools.

When planning your strength training routine, aim for balance. Include two to three sessions per week, allowing rest days in between to let your muscles recover and grow. Cover all muscle groups throughout the week to ensure a well-rounded approach and prevent overuse injuries. As you get stronger, gently increase the weight, resistance, or number of repetitions to continue challenging your muscles.

ESSENTIALS FOR STARTING YOUR STRENGTH TRAINING JOURNEY

1. Health Clearance:

- Schedule an appointment with your healthcare provider for a physical examination
- Discuss any existing health conditions and get clearance to start strength training

2. Goal Setting:

- Define clear, realistic strength training goals.
- Decide on the metrics you will use to track your progress.

3. Education and Planning:

- Research the basics of strength training, including techniques and safety tips.
- Choose a strength training program or routine suitable for beginners.
- Plan your workout schedule – decide how many days per week you will train.

4. Equipment and Space:

- Determine the necessary equipment (e.g., weights, resistance bands).
- If joining a gym, choose one that meets your needs and comfort level.
- If working out at home, set up a safe and comfortable space.

5. Exercise Selection:

- Select exercises that cover all major muscle groups.
- Ensure the routine includes both compound and isolation exercises.
- Learn the correct form for each exercise to avoid injury.

6. Nutrition and Hydration:

- Consult with a nutritionist or do research to understand your nutritional needs.
- Plan your meals and snacks to support your strength training and recovery.
- Stay hydrated by drinking water before, during, and after workouts.

7. Warm-up and Cool-down:

- Incorporate a 5-10 minute warm-up before starting your strength training.
- Include a cool-down period with stretching to aid recovery.

8. Tracking and Adjusting:

- Keep a workout log to track exercises, weights, sets, and reps.
- Regularly review your progress and adjust your program as needed.

9. Recovery and Rest:

- Schedule rest days to allow your muscles to recover.
- Pay attention to your body's signals and rest when needed.

10. Support System:

- Find a workout buddy, join a community, or hire a personal trainer for motivation and support.

This checklist is your roadmap to starting your strength training journey. Follow these steps to ensure you're well-prepared and set up for success in your new fitness routine.

As we navigate our golden years, embracing strength training is like lighting a path to maintaining and enhancing our physical capabilities. It's about building a foundation of strength that supports our independence, metabolism, and overall well-being. The journey involves gradual progress, thoughtful changes, and celebrating the inner strength we all possess.

Yoga and Flexibility: Enhancing Your Fasting Experience

Yoga is rooted in rich traditions and wisdom that harmonizes our mental and physical states. This harmonization is particularly beneficial when paired with the principles of IF, which advocate for a mindful approach to eating and living.

Think of yoga not just as exercise but as a symphony of movements, breathwork, and meditation. This unique combination enhances our well-being in so many ways. It helps us become more flexible, strengthens our muscles, and improves our posture, transforming our physical experience. But yoga does more than that; it steadies our thoughts and soothes our minds, teaching us to breathe through life's challenges quickly and clearly.

Imagine how yoga's blend of movement and breathwork prepares us for more profound relaxation, alleviates stress, and sharpens our mental focus—qualities that marry well with IF's reflective and purposeful nature.

As we age, flexibility becomes an increasingly important chapter in our lives, affecting our mobility and risk of injury. Regularly practicing yoga helps counteract the inevitable stiffness, making our daily movements smoother and safer. Think of it as greasing the hinges of a creaky door—yoga makes everything open and close a bit more smoothly.

On days when you're fasting, incorporating yoga can create a special kind of harmony. It's a way to stay active without draining your energy. Imagine starting your day with a gentle yoga session, setting a positive, grounded tone for your fasting hours, or unwinding in the evening with calming poses that prep you for a restorative sleep. Styles like Hatha or Yin are perfect for these days, with their slower pace and longer holds, nurturing your body without overwhelming it.

Now, let's weave mindfulness into this fabric—yoga and IF champion the art of being present and attuned to our bodies. On the yoga mat, we can dive inward, paying attention to our breath, feelings, and sensations without judgment. This awareness builds a stronger connection to our body's signals, aligning beautifully with the fasting ethos of responding to true hunger and satiety cues.

Carrying mindfulness from the mat into your day enhances the fasting experience, encouraging eating guided by internal cues rather than external pressures or fleeting emotions.

In essence, yoga is more than just physical practice; it's a pathway to a more prosperous, more attuned way of living. By integrating yoga into your fasting journey, you cultivate balance, flexibility, and mindfulness, enhancing your health and vitality both on and off the mat. It's not just about bending and stretching; it's about growing, understanding, and living more fully.

The Role of Cardio in Fat Loss and Heart Health

Cardiovascular exercise, often called cardio, is critical in your journey towards heart health and fat loss. Imagine cardio as your cheerleader for your heart, especially important for us ladies over 50. Our hearts need more love as we age, and cardio is a beautiful way to give them that care. After menopause, the risk of heart issues climbs, but here's the empowering part: regular cardio can significantly reduce this risk.

Think of cardio exercises like loving hugs for your heart. They get your blood pumping and ensure everything in your body gets the oxygen and nutrients needed. Cardio is more than just about losing weight; it's about strengthening your heart, lowering blood pressure, and balancing your cholesterol levels—sort of like tuning a musical instrument to play the sweetest melodies. Plus, when you engage in cardio, you're burning calories, which helps manage weight and fend off obesity, a sneaky culprit behind heart disease.

Now, the joy of cardio is that it comes in many flavors. Whether you enjoy a morning stroll, swimming laps at the pool, or cycling through the neighborhood, there's something for everyone. Start where you are; there's no rush. If you love walking, make it a part of your daily routine, gradually picking up the pace as you feel more comfortable. Swimming is like a gentle caress for your body, perfect for those who need a low-impact option. And cycling? It can be as leisurely or as challenging as you like. The goal is to find joy in movement, raising your heart rate and lifting your spirits.

Balancing cardio with strength training is like mixing the perfect cocktail: it gives you a blend of endurance, muscle tone, and bone health—all crucial elements, especially post-menopause. Aim to weave three days of cardio with two days of strength training into your week. This combo ensures you work on your heart and weight, build strength, and protect your bones.

Now, let's chat about intensity. It's all about finding that sweet spot where you're pushing yourself but not overdoing it. The 'talk test' is simple: if you can chat during your workout but can't belt out a song, you're likely at a moderate, manageable pace. And on fasting days, listen to your body – it's okay to dial down the intensity to match your energy levels. Remember, it's about supporting your body, not pushing it to extremes.

By incorporating cardio into your life, you're not just working out; you're creating a foundation for a vibrant, healthy future. Try different activities, mix strength training, and monitor your workout intensity. It's about building a lifestyle that keeps your heart happy, your body strong, and your spirit uplifted. Here's to moving, grooving, and loving our hearts more daily!

Creating a Balanced Exercise Routine

Your routine should be as diverse, adaptable, and personal as your favorite songs, blending strength, cardio, and flexibility to enrich your well-being and keep you resilient and vibrant.

Think of strength training as powerful ballads, building muscle and supporting your bones. Then there's cardio, your upbeat tracks, improving your heart's health and weight management. And don't forget about your smooth, calming songs – flexibility exercises – that increase your movement range and reduce injury risks.

Here's how to blend these into your weekly rhythm:

- **Strength Training**: Perform exercises that challenge your major muscle groups, like squats or push-ups, using whatever tools you have, such as body weight, free weights, or resistance bands.

- **Cardio Training**: Dedicate time to activities that raise your heart rate – maybe a dance, a swim, or a cycle, depending on what tunes into your mood.

- **Flexibility and Balance**: Add yoga or Pilates to stretch out and soothe your muscles, wrapping up your workouts like a gentle cooldown song.

Here's a sample of a weekly routine:

- **Monday**: Focus on lower-body strength.

- **Tuesday**: Pick up the pace with some cardio.

- **Wednesday**: Stretch and strengthen with yoga or Pilates.

- **Thursday**: Rest or light stretching – everyone needs a quiet interlude.

- **Friday**: Pump up the volume on upper-body strength.

- **Saturday**: Your choice of cardio – what's your weekend anthem?

- **Sunday**: Gentle activity, like a leisurely swim or a walk, to refresh.

Remember, this is just a template. Feel free to shuffle it around to suit your life's tempo.

Now, tuning this to your fitness level is critical:

- **Beginners**: Ease into it with gentler tunes, focusing on getting the moves right.

- **Intermediate**: Amp up with interval training or varied strength workouts.

- **Advanced**: Go for challenging rhythms with HIIT or intricate yoga poses.

Always listen to your body's feedback and adjust the volume accordingly. And if health concerns have you skipping tracks, reach out to a fitness professional to create a playlist that's just right for you.

But here's the chorus of our song: consistency. Regular, steady beats of moderate exercise will carry you further than occasional bursts of high intensity. It's about setting a pace you can keep up with and making it a fixed part of your daily schedule, like your favorite coffee or evening wind-down routine.

- **Set Achievable Goals**: Like crafting the perfect playlist, pick workouts that fit your lifestyle and keep you coming back for more.

- **Plan Ahead**: Schedule your exercise like important meetings – they are with you.

- **Track Your Progress**: Keep a log like a music diary. What made you feel good? What got you pumped?

YOUR WORKOUT WEEK PLANNED OUT

WEEK OF

Monday

- Morning: Fasted Cardio - 30 minutes walking or jogging
- Post-Workout Meal: Protein-rich breakfast within 1 hour after exercising.
- Tip: Stay hydrated, drink water or herbal tea before your workout.

Tuesday

- Afternoon: Strength Training - Full body (45 minutes)
- Post-Workout Meal: Balanced meal with protein, carbs, and fats, 1-2 hours post-exercise
- Tip: Focus on form and breathing.

Wednesday

- Evening: Yoga or Pilates - 1 hour
- Pre-Workout Meal: Light snack 30 minutes before, if within eating window
- Tip: Use this day for recovery and flexibility.

Thursday

- Morning: High-Intensity Interval Training (HIIT) - 30 minutes
- Post-Workout Meal: Refuel with a hearty meal, within your eating window
- Tip: Ensure you get enough sleep the night before.

Friday

- Afternoon: Leisure Activity (swimming, cycling, etc.) - 45 minutes
- Post-Workout Meal: Snack or meal depending on your fasting schedule
- Tip: End the workweek with something fun and less structured.

Saturday

- Morning or Afternoon: Active Recovery - Light walk, stretching, or foam rolling
- Meals: Follow your fasting schedule, eat light if you're not feeling hungry
- Tip: Listen to your body, rest if needed.

Sunday

- Rest Day
- Meals: Plan and prepare meals for the coming week
- Tip: Reflect on your week, adjust next week's schedule based on how you feel.

General Tips:
- Hydrate well every day, especially before and after workouts.
- Listen to your body: rest when needed and don't push through pain.
- Align your eating windows with your workout times for optimal energy and recovery.
- Remember, consistency is key. Adjust the intensity and type of workouts as needed.
- Keep track of your progress and how your body responds to different workouts and meal timings.

Crafting this balanced exercise routine isn't about sprinting to the finish line; it's about enjoying the journey, step by rhythmic step, towards a lifetime filled with health, strength, and joy. Let's create that playlist that keeps you dancing through life, feeling strong, balanced, and utterly in tune with yourself.

Listening to Your Body: Adjusting Workouts as Needed

Think of your body like a wise old friend who is always chatting with you and offering wisdom about when to push on and ease back. This is particularly important as we juggle the dance of fasting, feasting, and moving our bodies.

If you're constantly tired, irritable, having trouble sleeping, or finding your usual workouts suddenly daunting, your body might be pleading for a break. These are signs that it's time to embrace rest as part of your routine, allowing your muscles to heal and strengthen. Think of rest days and active recovery—like a leisurely walk or gentle yoga—as essential tunes in your life's playlist, keeping you flexible without overstraining.

Energy levels can be as unpredictable as the weather, influenced by our eating and fasting rhythms. On days when you're feeling more like a gentle stream than a roaring river, it's okay to adjust your workout's intensity or duration. There's harmony in aligning your exercise with your body's energy. If a morning run feels too much, maybe a brisk walk is just the right pace. Remember, your workout's quality counts, not necessarily how long or hard you go.

Let's talk about keeping injuries at bay. Warming up and cooling down aren't just opening and closing acts; they're key players in your fitness regime, prepping your body for the main event and helping it wind down afterward. Attention to your form, especially during weightlifting or complex routines, helps keep injuries offstage. Consider whether it fits you if a particular move consistently causes pain or discomfort.

Now, there will be days when the kindest thing you can do for your body is dial down your workout or skip it altogether. Illness, profound fatigue, or the beginnings of an injury are all signs of pulling back. Forcing yourself through pain or exhaustion isn't bravery; it can lead to more severe setbacks. Modifying your workout, like swapping a jog for a calming swim, can be a great middle ground.

It is crucial to understand the difference between the usual muscle burn after a good workout and signals of overdoing it. When you're unsure, lean on the side of caution. Opting for rest or a lighter activity can help you bounce back stronger and faster.

Recognizing the moments to push and pause in this ongoing conversation with your body is vital to a fulfilling fitness journey. It's about weaving together, fasting, feasting, and moving in a way that nourishes rather than depletes. You pave the way to lasting health and vitality by tuning in and responding thoughtfully. Let's cherish this dialogue, letting it guide us toward our most vibrant selves.

Overcoming Exercise Barriers: Tips for Staying Motivated

Think of your journey to regular exercise as navigating a maze—confusing and filled with obstacles. Still, you can turn it into an enjoyable adventure with the right mindset and strategies.

Identifying Personal Barriers: The first step is to uncover what's holding you back. Is it a packed schedule, a dip in motivation, or perhaps a dash of gym anxiety? By pinpointing these hurdles, you can tailor solutions to leap over them. If time is tight, why not weave exercise into your daily routine, like a brisk walk during lunch breaks or cycling to work? It's about spotlighting those hidden obstacles, making them smaller and less intimidating.

Why not keep a weekly diary of your exercise journey? Jot down moments when you skipped a workout and why. You'll start to see patterns and can plan your fitness adventure with these in mind.

Setting Achievable Goals: There's magic in setting just the right goals—challenging enough to spark your spirit but attainable sufficient to keep frustration at bay. Start with small victories, like a daily stroll or hitting a yoga mat a couple of times a week. As these small wins become part of your routine, they build a bridge to bigger dreams.

And remember, every big goal can be broken down into smaller, more manageable milestones. Celebrate each one to keep your motivation sky-high and to remind yourself of the progress you're making.

Finding Enjoyable Activities: Exercise should feel like a treat, not a chore. Dive into the search for activities that light a spark in you. If the open sky calls to you, maybe hiking or biking is your path. Or if the water's whisper beckons, perhaps swimming is your rhythm. There's a whole world of movement out there waiting for you to explore – try different things until you find the one that feels like it's meant just for you.

Building a Support System: Journeying with others can turn exercise from a solo slog into a shared celebration. Pair up with a friend who shares your fitness goals or join a community group that gets your heart racing in the best way. When your motivation dips, having someone to share the journey can be the nudge you need to lace up your sneakers and step out the door.

Connect with fitness groups in the real world and online to weave a net of support and encouragement. These communities can offer companionship, advice, and sometimes a gentle competition that keeps the spark of motivation alive.

A GUIDE TO OVERCOMING BARRIERS

This guide is designed to help you identify common barriers to exercise and provide you with practical solutions to overcome these obstacles. Use this as a reference whenever you need a motivational boost to maintain your fitness journey.

Barrier: Time Constraint
SOLUTION
- Plan Ahead: Schedule workouts as you would any important appointment.
- Micro Workouts: Integrate short, intense sessions of exercise throughout your day.
- Prioritize: Focus on quality, not quantity. Opt for shorter, more intense workouts when pressed for time.

Barrier: Lack of Motivation
SOLUTION
- Set Clear Goals: Define what you want to achieve and remind yourself why it's important.
- Find a Workout Buddy: Exercise with a friend to boost accountability and enjoyment.
- Reward Yourself: Set up a reward system for reaching your fitness milestones.

Barrier: Feeling Out of Place
SOLUTION
- Start Small: Begin with exercises that are within your comfort zone and gradually expand your horizons.
- Research: Learn about different workout routines and what to expect beforehand.
- Supportive Environment: Find a workout space where you feel comfortable and supported.

Barrier: Lack of Knowledge
SOLUTION
- Educate Yourself: Utilize online resources, books, or fitness apps to understand exercises and their proper forms.
- Hire a Trainer: Consider working with a professional to get personalized guidance and instruction.
- Join Classes: Participate in group classes where an instructor can provide direct feedback and support.

Barrier: Physical Discomfort or Pain
SOLUTION
- Consult a Professional: Speak with a healthcare provider to address pain or physical limitations.
- Modify Your Workout: Adjust exercises to accommodate any discomfort or use supportive gear.
- Warm-Up and Cool Down: Incorporate comprehensive warm-up and cool-down routines to prevent injury.

Barrier: Boredom
SOLUTION
- Mix It Up: Regularly change your workout routine to include a variety of activities.
- Try New Things: Experiment with different types of exercises, classes, or outdoor activities.
- Set New Challenges: Keep your workouts exciting by setting new goals and challenges.

Barrier: Weather Conditions
SOLUTION
- Be Prepared: Have indoor workout options ready for bad weather days.
- Dress Appropriately: Invest in proper gear for different weather conditions.
- Embrace Nature: When safe, use the weather to your advantage for new workout experiences.

Remember, every journey has its hurdles, but overcoming them makes you stronger. Keep this guide handy and refer to it whenever you're facing an obstacle in your fitness journey. Stay motivated, stay flexible, and keep pushing forward towards your health and fitness goals.

DISCOVER YOUR EXERCISE PERSONALITY

This brief questionnaire is designed to identify your exercise preferences and match you with physical activities you're likely to enjoy. Answer the following questions about your likes, dislikes, how you prefer to spend your free time, and your past experiences with physical activity. Based on your responses, we'll provide personalized suggestions to help you incorporate more movement into your life.

Social Preferences:

- I prefer to exercise alone; I find it more peaceful and productive.

- I enjoy exercising with a partner or in small groups; it's motivating and fun.

- I love being part of a class or team; the more, the merrier!

Activity Level:

- I prefer low-intensity activities; they're relaxing and easier to start.

- I enjoy moderate-intensity activities; they're engaging but not too exhausting.

- I love high-intensity activities; they're challenging and invigorating!

Indoors or Outdoors:

- I prefer indoor activities; they're convenient and weather-proof.

- I enjoy both; variety is the spice of life!

- I love outdoor activities; nature and fresh air are revitalizing!

Competition:

- I prefer non-competitive activities; I'm more focused on self-improvement.

- I enjoy light competition; it's motivating but not too serious.

- I love competition; it pushes me to perform at my best!

Routine vs. Variety:

- I prefer sticking to a routine; it's easier to follow and track progress.

- I enjoy a mix of routine and new activities; it keeps things interesting.

- I love trying new things; I'm always up for a new challenge!

Time of Day:

- I prefer morning workouts; they energize me for the day ahead.

- I enjoy afternoon or evening workouts; they're a great way to wind down.

- I'm flexible; I can fit in exercise anytime.

Suggestions:

- If you prefer solo, low-intensity, indoor activities, you might enjoy yoga, pilates, or swimming.

- If you enjoy group, high-intensity, outdoor activities, you might enjoy boot camps, cycling groups, or team sports.

- If you prefer a mix, you might benefit from a gym membership that offers various classes, or you could alternate between solo jogging and group dance classes.

The best type of exercise is the one you enjoy and can stick with in the long run. Use your exercise personality insights to explore new activities and find what works best for you. Keep experimenting until you find your perfect fit, and have fun on your journey to a more active lifestyle!

YOUR PERSONALIZED FITNESS BLUEPRINT

1 Assess Your Current Fitness Level

Baseline Assesment:
Record your current physical condition, including weight, body measurements, strength, and endurance levels. This might include how long you can jog, how many push-ups you can do, etc.

Health Check:
Consult with a healthcare provider if necessary to understand any limitations or precautions.

2 Define Clear, Achievable Goals

Set SMART Goals:
Ensure your fitness goals are Specific, Measurable, Achievable, Relevant, and Time-bound.

Prioritize:
Decide which goals are most important to you and focus on those first.

3 Choose Activities You Enjoy

Explore Options:
List physical activities you enjoy or might like to try, from walking or cycling to dance classes or yoga.

Variety:
Incorporate different types of exercise (aerobic, strength training, flexibility, and balance) to cover all aspects of fitness.

4 Create Your Workout Schedule

Plan Weekly:
Design a weekly routine that alternates between different types of exercise and includes rest days.

Be Realistic:
Make sure your workout times and durations fit comfortably into your daily schedule.

5 Build Your Support System

Find a Buddy:
Partner with a friend who has similar fitness goals or join a group to increase accountability.

Seek Professional Help:
Consider hiring a personal trainer or joining a class for additional guidance and motivation.

YOUR PERSONALIZED FITNESS BLUEPRINT

6 Equip Yourself

Baseline Assesment:
Record your current physical condition, including weight, body measurements, strength, and endurance levels. This might include how long you can jog, how many push-ups you can do, etc.

Health Check:
Consult with a healthcare provider if necessary to understand any limitations or precautions.

7 Start Your Fitness Journey

Begin Gradually:
Start with lighter, shorter sessions and gradually increase the intensity and duration.

Listen to Your Body:
Pay attention to how you feel during and after workouts and adjust as necessary.

8 Track Your Progress

Log Activities:
Record your workouts, including what you did and how you felt.

Review and Adjust:
Regularly review your progress towards your goals and make changes to your plan as needed.

9 Celebrate Achievements

Plan Weekly:
Recognize when you reach a goal or consistently follow your routine.

Reward Yourself:
Treat yourself to something you enjoy as a reward for your hard work.

10 Maintain and Update Your Plan

Stay Flexible:
Be prepared to adapt your blueprint as your fitness level, goals, or circumstances change.

Continuous Improvement:
Keep challenging yourself with new goals or different activities to stay motivated and progress.

Staying motivated to exercise regularly is a dynamic process with ups and downs. Navigating the fitness maze becomes less about the destination and more about enjoying each step, leap, and sprint. By understanding and overcoming your barriers, setting thoughtful goals, finding joy in movement, and embracing the journey with others, exercise transforms into a rewarding part of your daily life – a path to physical wellness, happiness, and fulfillment.

The Connection Between Physical Activity and Hormonal Balance

Your body operates through a complex system where hormones regulate mood and metabolism. Physical activity plays a crucial role in this system, helping to keep your hormones balanced and ensuring your body functions smoothly. When we engage in regular exercise, we support our body's systems in working together effectively, leading to better overall health and well-being.

The Magic of Exercise and Endorphins: Imagine walking briskly or enjoying a refreshing swim. This movement triggers the release of endorphins, our body's natural mood lifters. These biochemicals ease the pain and sprinkle joy into our day as a natural buffer to life's stresses. It's like finding a serene spot during chaos, reminding us that taking care of our body is taking care of our mind.

Exercise Meets Menopause: The journey through menopause can be a rollercoaster, with its ups and downs manifesting as hot flashes or mood changes—exercise steps in here as a comforting friend. Regular movement, particularly aerobic activities, can ease the heat of hot flashes, while gentle practices like yoga offer a peaceful retreat for the mind, smoothing out the emotional waves. It's about tuning our exercise routines to the rhythm of our changing bodies, providing a personalized cushion against these shifts.

The Hormonal Response to Movement: Our body's hormone levels ebb and flow in response to how we move. Take cortisol, our stress-signaling hormone; its levels can peak with intense activity, but find a balanced rhythm with regular, moderate exercise. Physical activity also polishes our insulin sensitivity, safeguarding our metabolic health. This dance of hormones underlines the importance of choosing exercises that suit our body's needs and journey, particularly as we navigate life's different stages.

Crafting Your Exercise Blueprint for Hormonal Health: When we tailor our exercise routine to support our hormonal balance, especially during life phases like menopause, it's fine-tuning our internal orchestra to play harmoniously. Consider these steps:

- **Moderate Aerobic Exercise**: Include moderate aerobic exercise like brisk walking or swimming in your weekly routine. These activities keep the heart happy and hormones in check without overwhelming the body.

- **Strength Training**: Sprinkle in some strength training a few times weekly. This helps combat muscle loss that comes with age, supports your bones, and keeps your weight healthy.

- **Flexibility and Balance**: Do yoga or Pilates to stay limber and grounded. These practices deepen your body awareness and bring peace, like a quiet lullaby for your nervous system.

- **Listen to Your Body**: This is your journey; how you feel is your guide. If certain activities stir up menopause symptoms or feel too heavy, it's okay to switch gears. Perhaps choose a gentler form of movement or a shorter routine on days when your energy whispers for rest.

Incorporating varied exercises that favor hormonal balance can shift how we experience our bodies during menopause and beyond. It's about making empowered choices that bolster our physical and emotional health. By listening to our body's whispers and adjusting our fitness melodies, we can glide through the hormonal waves of menopause with poise and strength, keeping our well-being as the show's star.

Tracking Progress: Beyond the Scale

In fitness and health, particularly as we move beyond age 50, it becomes increasingly important to look at the broader picture of our achievements rather than focusing solely on the numbers on a scale. Understanding and acknowledging the variety of ways fitness success can manifest is essential for a balanced and fulfilling journey.

Measuring Success Differently: Fitness success is not just about weight. It includes gains in strength, such as lifting heavier weights or doing more repetitions, which is crucial for maintaining muscle and overall health. Increased energy levels throughout the day and enhanced well-being, including better mood and lower stress, are significant progress markers. These aspects contribute to a comprehensive view of your health improvements.

Non-Scale Victories: Many milestones in your fitness journey have nothing to do with weight. For example, fitting into previously tight clothes can be a clear sign of your progress, reflecting changes in your body's shape and composition. Overcoming challenges in workouts or activities that were once out of reach showcases your increased physical abilities and mental determination. Improvements in flexibility and mobility, which make everyday activities easier, also mark significant progress.

Long-term Health Markers: Exercise has a profound impact on long-term health markers that can offer insights into the more profound benefits of your regimen. These include lower blood pressure, vital for heart health, improved cholesterol levels, and better blood sugar control. These changes are essential for long-term health and well-being and offer a more meaningful measure of success than scale weight alone.

Reflecting on Personal Growth: The journey of incorporating regular exercise into your life is as much about personal development as it is about physical changes. Regular activity can boost your confidence and self-esteem, reflecting your ability to meet and surpass goals. It also builds resilience, helping you to overcome challenges and bounce back stronger. Moreover, finding joy in movement, whether through dance, yoga, or walking, marks a significant shift toward viewing exercise as a rewarding part of your life.

FITNESS PROGRESS TRACKER

DATE: / /

S M T W T F S

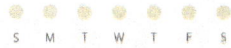

Goals & Achievements

Short-Term Goals (This month)

Long-Term Goals (3 monts, 6 months, 1 year)

Achievements

MOOD

ANGRY   TIRED   SAD   HAPPY   EXCITED

NOTES (Triggers, improvements, correlating activities)

HEALTH MARKERS

Weight: _____

Resting Heart Rate _____

Blood Pressure _____

Other Relevant Markers) _____

WORKOUTS

Type of Exercise (e.g. Cardio, Yoga):

Duration: _____

Intensity (Light, Moderate, High):

Energy Level (Scale of 1 -10)

Notes (Factors affecting energy:

STRENGTH GAINS

Exercise (e.g. Squats):

Weight Lifted:

Reps & Sets:

Progress Notes (Improvements, challenges): _____

PERSONAL REFLECTIONS

Reflections on progress (Overall progress, how you're feeling about your fitness journey)

Challenges faced and how they were overcome

Adjustments to goals or methods (Changes to routine, goals)

We can appreciate the full benefits of an active lifestyle by shifting our focus from the scale to a broader view of progress and well-being. Celebrating each step forward reinforces the importance of our efforts and contributes to a more meaningful, health-centered life. This approach helps deepen our connection to our bodies and emphasizes the significance of nurturing our health at every stage of life.

Recovery and Rest: Essential Elements of Your Fitness Routine

Recovery and rest are crucial elements of any fitness routine, particularly as we get older, and our bodies need more time to heal and rejuvenate after exercise. Understanding the importance of these aspects can make a significant difference in your fitness success and longevity.

The Importance of Recovery

Your body needs time to repair and strengthen itself after a workout. This rest period is essential for muscle repair, especially after strength training, which causes tiny tears in muscle fibers. Recovery isn't just about physical benefits; it helps prevent mental burnout and maintain motivation and enjoyment in your fitness journey.

Types of Recovery:

- **Active Recovery**: This involves light activities such as walking, gentle stretching, or yoga, which help to keep the blood flowing and reduce muscle stiffness and soreness after more intense workout days. It's a way to stay moving without overexerting yourself.

- **Passive Recovery**: You allow your body to rest without structured physical activity. Deep rest is vital for your body's healing process, helping you recover deeper and prepare for the next workout.

Nutrition and Hydration for Recovery

What you eat and drink significantly affects how quickly and effectively your body recovers after exercise. Including protein-rich foods in your post-workout meal helps with muscle repair, while anti-inflammatory foods can reduce swelling and soreness. Staying hydrated, particularly with water or sometimes electrolyte-infused drinks, is also crucial for adequate recovery.

Listening to Your Body

Paying attention to your body's signals is essential. If you feel unusually tired or sore or notice a decreased performance, these could be signs that your body needs more rest. Quality sleep is also critical to recovery; getting enough rest each night can significantly improve your fitness and health.

Incorporating proper recovery and rest into your fitness routine is as important as the workouts. By respecting your body's need for rest, you can avoid injuries, improve your performance, and find more joy and vitality in your fitness journey. Remember, fitness is not just about pushing your limits; it's also about allowing your body the time it needs to rest, heal, and grow stronger.

Celebrating Milestones and Setting New Goals

In our journey through fitness and well-being, we must stop and recognize the milestones we've reached. Celebrating these achievements motivates us and reminds us of our progress. It's essential to take a moment to acknowledge every success, whether completing a run, achieving a new yoga pose, or maintaining a regular workout schedule. These milestones are significant and worthy of celebration.

Recognizing Achievements

Celebrating your successes is essential for maintaining motivation and reinforcing your commitment to a healthy lifestyle. Here's how you can honor your progress:

- Keep a record of your achievements, creating a physical or digital board to see your progress.

- Share your successes with friends or family, drawing on their support and encouragement.

Celebrate Your Victories

These platforms can provide valuable insights into designing user-friendly interfaces, engaging community features, and practical tracking tools for health and wellness goals. Each has unique elements that could inspire features in your Victory Vistas platform, especially around community engagement, personal tracking, and shared experiences.

MyFitnessPal: This well-known app tracks diet and exercise and helps users monitor their nutrition and physical activity levels. It includes features for logging food intake and exercise and connecting with friends for support and motivation.

Fitbit Community: Part of the Fitbit app, this feature allows users to join groups, participate in challenges, and share their fitness achievements with others. It's a great example of integrating community support with personal health tracking.

Strava: A social network for athletes, Strava primarily tracks cycling and running exercises using GPS data. It includes features for sharing routes, joining clubs, and participating in challenges, making it a community-driven solid platform.

Headspace Community: While Headspace is primarily a meditation and mindfulness app, it also includes a community aspect where users can share their experiences and support each other's mental health journeys.

SparkPeople: Offers a comprehensive suite of health tools, including a food diary, exercise log, and health community. Users can track their progress towards their health goals and engage with others for support and motivation.

Habitica: A unique platform that turns personal goals and to-do lists into a role-playing game. Users can join parties, complete quests, and earn rewards alongside others, making habit formation fun and social.

Peloton Community: Beyond its fitness equipment, Peloton has a strong community component where users can join live classes together, compete on leaderboards, and connect with other members.

Noom: Known for its psychological approach to weight loss and habit change, Noom also includes a community aspect where users can support each other, share successes, and discuss challenges.

Calm Community: Similar to Headspace, Calm is a meditation app with more community features. It allows users to share stories and support each other's mindfulness practices.

PatientsLikeMe: Although more focused on chronic illness, this platform allows users to track their health, find others with similar conditions, and share their experiences and treatments, providing a solid example of a support-based community.

Setting New Fitness Goals

As you reach each milestone, consider what new goals you can set. This keeps your fitness journey exciting and challenging:

- Reflect on the parts of your fitness routine that you enjoy the most and think about how to expand on these areas.

- Make your new goals clear and measurable. Decide what you want to achieve next, whether lifting weights, running longer further, or trying a different class.

Reflecting on Your Journey

Taking time to reflect helps you appreciate the full extent of your progress. It's not just about physical changes but also about the mental and emotional growth you've experienced:

- Maintain a journal of your fitness journey, noting how you felt at different points and what you've learned.

Planning for the Future

Looking ahead and planning your future fitness goals is an exciting step. This involves setting new targets and considering how your interests and needs might change:

- Outline your short-term and long-term fitness goals, breaking them down into smaller steps.

- Be flexible with your planning, allowing your goals to evolve with you.

REFLECT ON YOUR JOURNEY

DATE: / /

S M T W T F S

PHYSICAL REFLECTIONS

Recall a time before your fitness routine. How would your past self react to the physical activities you can perform now?

How has your physical strength and endurance changed since you began your fitness journey?

What physical achievements are you most proud of, and what do they mean about your overall health?

REFLECT ON YOUR JOURNEY

DATE: /   /

S   M   T   W   T   F   S

MENTAL AND EMOTIONAL REFLECTIONS

How has your mental health been affected by your fitness routine?

Can you identify any stress levels or anxiety changes since starting your fitness journey? What activities have had the most significant impact?

Reflect on a moment during your fitness journey where you felt a strong emotional response (joy, pride, frustration). What triggered this response, and what did it teach you?

REFLECT ON YOUR JOURNEY

DATE: / /

S M T W T F S

SELF-PERCEPTION AND CONFIDENCE

How has your self-perception changed since you began your fitness routine?

Are there activities or challenges you now approach confidently that previously intimidated you?

How does your current fitness level align with the identity or self-image you wish to cultivate?

REFLECT ON YOUR JOURNEY

DATE: /   /

S   M   T   W   T   F   S

LIFESTYLE AND HABITS

How has your daily routine or lifestyle changed to accommodate your fitness goals?

Reflect on your most consistent fitness habits. How did you develop them, and how do they serve you?

Reflect on your most consistent fitness habits. How did you develop them, and how do they serve you?

REFLECT ON YOUR JOURNEY

DATE: / /

S M T W T F S

HOLISTIC HEALTH AND WELLBEING

How do you feel your physical fitness has influenced your overall health and well-being?

Reflect on balancing your physical, mental, and emotional health. How has this balance shifted since starting your fitness journey?

What are the most significant lessons you've learned about yourself and your health through your fitness experiences?

Recognizing our achievements and setting new goals are vital in our fitness journey. They remind us of our progress and help propel us towards new challenges. As we move forward, we should do so with curiosity, openness to change, and a solid commitment to our health and well-being. This approach helps us confidently continue our journey, armed with the knowledge and experiences we've gathered.

Chapter 4

Making IF Work for You

Your health is what you make of it. Everything you do and think
either adds to the vitality, energy, and spirit you possess or takes
away from it. Ann Wigmore

I magine starting your day with clarity and ending it with a sense of accomplishment, all while nurturing your body in a way that feels right for you.
That's the promise of integrating IF into your life, not as a rigid system but as
a flexible framework tailored to fit the rhythm of your daily activities. It's like
finding the perfect pair of jeans; everything else falls into place when it works
right. This chapter offers practical strategies to blend IF with your personal and
professional life seamlessly, ensuring it enhances rather than hinders your daily
routine.

Integrating IF into Your Daily Life

Let's begin by tailoring IF to fit seamlessly into your schedule. Take a moment
to review your week—consider your fixed commitments and the times you have
some flexibility. It's essential that your fasting schedule feels like a natural part of
your day, not something that disrupts your routine. If your mornings are usually

busy, your fasting could start after breakfast. If family dinners are important, ensure your eating window accommodates these precious moments. Remember, IF methods, such as the 16/8 or 5/2 approaches, are flexible. Pick the method that meshes well with your lifestyle.

Establishing Routines and Rituals

Simple rituals can beautifully mark the beginning and end of your fasting periods. For example, you might start your day with a calming cup of herbal tea to signify the start of fasting or end it with a nourishing meal to close the window. Over time, these practices will naturally become part of your daily rhythm, providing stability and meaning to your fasting journey.

Embracing Flexibility

Accept that life comes with its twists and turns. There will be days when following your fasting schedule feels effortless and others when it feels challenging. It's okay to be flexible. Adjusting your fasting for the day is OK if something unexpected, like a social brunch, comes up. What's important is the consistency of your pattern over time—not adhering rigidly to a schedule every single day. Use IF as a positive addition to your life, not a restriction.

Utilizing Technology and Tools

In today's digital world, various apps and tools can help support your fasting journey. They can track your fasting windows, remind you to stay hydrated, and even connect you with a community of people who are also fasting. Take some time to explore these options and find the tools that suit your needs, adding a layer of convenience to your fasting practice.

TOP APPS AND TOOLS

ZERO - FASTING TRACKER

- **Features**: User-friendly fasting timer, personalized fasting plans, and insights into your fasting habits.

- **Unique Selling Point:** Offers various fasting windows to choose from and tracks your fasting history.

FASTIC - FASTING APP

- **Features:** Fasting timer, hydration tracker, step counter, and weight tracking.

- **Unique Selling Point:** Includes educational resources to help you understand the science behind IF.

LIFE FASTING TRACKER

- **Features**: Fasting timer, social support through community features, and progress tracking.

- **Unique Selling Point:** You can track ketone levels and glucose and connect with friends for motivation.

MYFITNESSPAL

- **Features:** Comprehensive food database for nutritional tracking, barcode scanner, and calorie counter.

- **Unique Selling Point**: Integrates diet tracking with exercise to provide a complete picture of your health.

WATERMINDER

- **Features:** Hydration reminders, customizable water intake goals, and historical consumption logs.

- **Unique Selling Point**: Provides detailed hydration statistics and reminders to ensure you stay hydrated.

TOP APPS AND TOOLS

DAILYDO – PLANNER & HABIT TRACKER

- **Features:** Habit tracking, daily planner, and task manager.

- **Unique Selling Point:** Helps you build and track new habits, such as regular eating windows and fasting periods.

EAT THIS MUCH - MEAL PLANNER

- **Features:** Automatic meal planner, grocery list generator, and calorie counter.

- **Unique Selling Point:** Creates personalized meal plans based on your dietary preferences, budget, and schedule.

HEADSPACE - MEDITATION & SLEEP

- **Features:** Guided meditations, sleep sounds, and mindfulness exercises.

- **Unique Selling Point:** Offers mindfulness practices to help manage hunger and stress while fasting.

CRONOMETER

- **Features:** Detailed nutritional tracking, biometric data logging, and health reports.

- **Unique Selling Point:** Allows micronutrient tracking to ensure you get all necessary nutrients within your eating window.

INSIGHT TIMER - MEDITATION APP

- **Features:** Free library of meditations, music for relaxation, and sleep aids.

- **Unique Selling Point:** Wide range of meditation topics, including ones for stress, sleep, and self-love, supporting mental well-being during fasting.

FIND YOUR FASTING FIT

Take this personalized quiz to determine which IF method — 16/8, 5:2, or Eat-Stop-Eat — best fits your unique lifestyle, habits, and goals. Answer the following questions based on your current lifestyle, eating habits, and how you manage your health and social commitments.

1

How would you describe your eating patterns?

A) I prefer eating smaller meals and snacks throughout the day.
B) I'm comfortable with having fewer, more substantial meals.
C) I can go for days without eating much but prefer larger meals.

2

How flexible is your daily schedule in terms of meal timing?

A) I am very flexible; I can easily adjust my meal times.
B) Somewhat flexible; I can plan my eating around fixed points in my day.
C) I am not very flexible; I prefer more traditional meal times.

3

What's your main goal for trying intermittent fasting?

A) To improve overall health and wellness.
B) To lose weight in a manageable way.
C) To challenge myself and see significant results.

4

How do you manage hunger?

A) I find it challenging and prefer not to feel too hungry.
B) I'm okay feeling a bit hungry if I know my next meal is coming.
C) I can handle significant hunger and focus on other things.

5

How do you handle social eating situations (e.g., parties, dinners out)?

A) I frequently attend social events and prefer not to restrict my eating.
B) I can skip some social eating occasions or choose lighter options.
C) I'm comfortable not eating at social events if it's a fasting day.

6

How do you feel about tracking your food intake and calories?

A) I prefer not to count calories but can track my eating times.
B) I'm okay with some tracking as long as it's not every day.
C) I'm willing to track my calorie intake closely on certain days.

7

What approach to dietary change feels most sustainable to you?

A) Gradual changes that fit seamlessly into my current lifestyle.
B) Moderate changes that require some planning but are not too restrictive.
C) More significant changes that might be challenging but offer clear rules.

FIND YOUR FASTING FIT

RESULTS:

Mostly As:

16/8 Method – This flexible approach, involving 16 hours of fasting followed by an 8-hour eating window, might suit your lifestyle and preference for not feeling too hungry. It allows for regular meals and snacks during your eating period, giving you control over your eating habits.

Mostly Bs:

5:2 Method – With the 5:2 approach, you usually eat five days a week and reduce calorie intake on two non-consecutive days. This could align with your willingness to track some meals and manage moderate hunger while enjoying most social events without restriction.

Mostly Cs:

Eat-Stop-Eat – This might be the best fit for you if you can handle significant hunger and are okay with abstaining from food for 24 hours, once or twice a week. It's suited for those who prefer clear rules and are willing to forego eating during social events on fasting days.

Remember, these are just guidelines based on your answers. It's essential to consult with a healthcare professional before starting any new diet plan, especially one that includes fasting.

Incorporating IF into your routine can be straightforward and rewarding with careful planning, the right attitude, and a readiness to adapt. By crafting a fasting schedule that acknowledges your commitments, embedding meaningful rituals into your day, staying flexible, and using available technology, IF can transform from a mere diet into a sustainable, enjoyable lifestyle tailored just for you.

Managing Social Events and Dining Out

Managing social events and dining out while keeping up with IF requires careful planning and effective communication. It's all about finding a balance that allows you to enjoy social occasions and your health goals without feeling overwhelmed.

Pre-Planning Strategies

Planning ahead to incorporate social events into your fasting routine is essential. Note upcoming gatherings and adjust your fasting schedule accordingly. You might need to start your fast earlier or break it later to fit in with your social commitments. Keeping a calendar of events alongside your fasting schedule can help you stay organized and make necessary adjustments.

Navigating Menu Choices

You don't have to stress finding the perfect meal when dining out. Most restaurants offer a variety of options that can align with your nutritional needs. Before you go, take a moment to look over the menu online. Choose dishes that fit within your eating window and dietary preferences. If you're about to start your fasting period, opt for lighter options like salads or grilled vegetables. To break your fast, lean proteins and complex carbohydrates can provide a balanced refuel. Don't hesitate to ask for modifications to suit your needs – chefs are usually happy to accommodate.

Communicating with Friends and Family

Being open about your fasting lifestyle with loved ones can lead to understanding and support. Explain the basics of IF and why it's important to you. Emphasize that while you value your time together, you're also committed to choices that support your well-being. Most friends and family will respect your dedication once they understand how it benefits you.

Enjoying Moderation

Find a balance between enjoying social events and sticking to your fasting goals. Allow yourself to indulge moderately, even if it falls outside your eating window or dietary preferences. This approach fosters a healthy relationship with food, where you can enjoy the moment without guilt. Remember, IF is about consistency, not perfection. Aim to follow your plan most of the time, but allow flexibility to enjoy life's special moments.

Social events and dining out while IF do not have to be daunting. By planning, communicating effectively, and practicing moderation, you can enjoy the best of both worlds without sacrificing your health goals. These strategies help integrate fasting into your lifestyle, making it a sustainable and enjoyable practice.

Emotional Eating and IF: Finding Balance

It's essential to understand that managing emotional eating goes beyond sheer willpower. It involves recognizing what triggers our eating habits and establishing a balanced approach that honors our physical and emotional health.

Identifying Emotional Eating Triggers

The first step is identifying what prompts you to seek comfort in food. This could be due to various emotions like stress, boredom, or sadness. I recommend keeping a diary to track your food intake and emotions. Start with simple notes on your smartphone or a notebook. Try to capture as much context as possible: what you eat, the time, preceding events, and how you feel. Soon, you'll start noticing patterns and triggers previously under your radar.

Mindfulness and Awareness

Mindfulness is critical in distinguishing between the sudden, urgent cravings of emotional hunger and the gradual onset of physical hunger. When you feel an urge to eat, pause and ask yourself if you're hungry or just trying to feed an emotion. Even a brief pause can help break the cycle of emotional eating. You could also try deep breathing or meditation to help center yourself before making a food choice. If emotions drive your hunger, think about other activities, like a walk or a warm bath, that could meet your emotional needs.

Coping Mechanisms

Developing healthy ways to cope with stress and emotions that don't involve eating is crucial. This could mean turning to yoga or exercise to relieve stress and boost your mood or engaging in creative hobbies like painting or writing to provide emotional fulfillment without eating. Find what works for you and makes you feel good without relying on food.

Support Systems

A robust support system can significantly impact your journey. Connect with friends, family, or online communities who understand the challenges of IF and can provide support and advice. Consider joining forums or social media groups to share experiences and strategies with others facing similar challenges. An accountability buddy who knows your fasting goals and schedule can also be invaluable in reminding you of your commitments when you're tempted by emotional eating.

Incorporating these strategies into your IF routine can help ensure a balanced approach that nourishes your body and respects your emotional well-being. By acknowledging emotional triggers, practicing mindfulness, developing healthy coping

Mechanisms and leveraging your support network, you set yourself on a sustainable path that aligns with your lifestyle and goals.

The Power of Community and Sharing Your Journey

Engaging with the right support network can significantly enhance your IF journey, transforming it from a solo venture into a collective experience. A community of individuals who share your goals can offer encouragement, exchange insights, and celebrate your achievements with you, making the entire process more manageable and enjoyable.

> *REAL JOURNEY: Marrianne, 62, was skeptical about IF but decided to try it after her doctor's recommendation. The early days were challenging, filled with irritability and sleep disturbances. Marriane almost quit but chose instead to seek support from fasting communities online. This interaction helped her tweak her fasting approach to include lighter activities like yoga during fasting hours, which significantly improved her experience. Marriane's story illustrates how community support can transform a harrowing journey into a manageable one.*

Finding a Supportive Community

To find a community that meets your needs, consider what type of support you seek. Many online forums and social media groups focus on IF when you can share experiences, ask questions, and celebrate successes. Don't overlook local health or wellness groups, which may hold seminars or meet-ups. Actively participating by asking questions, sharing your journey, and supporting others is crucial. This engagement creates a network of mutual support to lean on during tough times.

A GUIDE TO ONLINE & LOCAL COMMUNITIES

Joining a fasting community can provide motivation, accountability, and valuable insights as you navigate your fasting journey. Whether online or local, these communities can be a source of immense support and encouragement. Here's how to find your fasting tribe and make the most of these groups.

Finding Online Fasting Communities:

Meetup Groups:
- Use Meetup.com to find local fasting or health-oriented groups. Attend a few meetings to see if the group's focus aligns with your interests and goals.

Local Health and Wellness Centers:
- Inquire at local gyms, yoga studios, or wellness centers if they know of any fasting groups or are interested in starting one.

Start Your Group:
- If you can't find a local group, consider starting your own. Use social media or community bulletin boards to invite others interested in fasting to join.

What to Look for in a Fasting Community:

Positive and Supportive Environment:
- Look for groups that foster positivity, encouragement, and respectful discussion.

Knowledge Sharing:
- A good fasting community should be informative, sharing valuable tips, articles, and resources to help you learn more about fasting.

Diverse Experiences:
- Communities with members at different stages of their fasting journey can provide a broader perspective and more comprehensive advice.

Privacy and Safety:
- Ensure the community respects privacy and provides a safe space for sharing personal experiences.

Active Participation:
- A vibrant community should have regular posts, updates, and discussions to keep members engaged and supported.

A GUIDE TO ONLINE & LOCAL COMMUNITIES

Engaging with Your Fasting Community:

Introduce Yourself:
- Share your fasting goals, experiences, and what you hope to gain from the community.

Ask Questions:
- Don't hesitate to ask for advice or clarification on fasting topics you're unsure about.

Share Your Experiences:
- Contributing your own stories and insights can help others and foster a sense of camaraderie.

Respect Different Approaches:
- Remember that fasting can look different for everyone. Respect and learn from the diversity of approaches within your community.

Stay Active and Supportive:
- Regular participation can help you stay motivated and support others on their fasting journeys.

Finding your fasting tribe can significantly enhance your fasting experience, providing you with a network of like-minded individuals who can offer support, motivation, and advice. Whether online or in-person, taking the time to find the right community can lead to lasting friendships and a more enjoyable and successful fasting journey.

BUILDING YOUR SUPPORT SYSTEM

This guide is designed to assist you in developing a robust and supportive relationship with an accountability partner. Following these steps, you can establish a partnership fostering mutual growth and achievement.

Identify a Potential Accountability Partner

- Shared Goals: Seek individuals with similar objectives. Are you both aiming for professional advancement, healthier lifestyles, or mastering a new skill?

- Commitment Level: Find someone with a matching level of commitment. Is this individual as determined as you are to achieve their goals?

- Compatibility: Ensure your schedules, communication styles, and personalities complement each other.

- Motivation: Choose a partner who motivates you. Do they inspire you to be your best self?

Connecting with Your Potential Partner

- Introduction: Reach out with a clear and friendly message. Share a bit about yourself, your goals, and why you seek an accountability partner.

- Initial Meeting: Arrange a meeting (in-person or online) to discuss your goals and expectations and see if you click.

- Set Boundaries: Talk about your boundaries and preferences upfront to ensure mutual respect and understanding.

BUILDING YOUR SUPPORT SYSTEM

Questions to Ask a Potential Accountability Partner

- What are your main goals for the upcoming months?

- How do you plan to achieve your goals?

- What do you expect from an accountability partnership?

- How often would you like to check in, and through what means?

- What challenges have you faced while trying to achieve similar goals?

- How do you handle setbacks, and how can I best support you during those times?

Strategies for a Successful Accountability Partnership

- Consistent Check-ins: Agree on a regular schedule for updates and encourage each other.

- Honest Communication: Be transparent about your progress, challenges, and feelings.

- Constructive Feedback: Give and receive helpful, respectful, and constructive feedback.

- Celebrate Success: Acknowledge both your and your partner's achievements.

- Adapt and Reevaluate: Be willing to adjust your strategies and goals as needed.

- Supportive Environment: Create a judgment-free zone where you feel comfortable sharing successes and setbacks.

BUILDING YOUR SUPPORT SYSTEM

Maintaining the Relationship

- Mutual Respect: Always treat each other with respect and understanding.

- Flexibility: Life happens. Be understanding if your partner needs to reschedule or adjust goals.

- Problem-solving: If issues arise, address them directly and work together to find solutions.

- Gratitude: Regularly appreciate your partner's support and dedication.

Fostering Mutual Growth

- An effective accountability partnership is built on mutual respect, open communication, and shared commitment to growth. By selecting the right partner and employing these strategies, you can create a support system that propels both of you toward your goals. Remember, the journey is about progress, not perfection; having someone to share it with can make all the difference.

Engaging with a supportive community or accountability partner can enrich your IF experience. It turns an individual endeavor into a collective adventure, where everyone's contributions help build a network of support and encouragement. By sharing your story and learning from the group's collective wisdom, you make the path of IF more sustainable and profoundly fulfilling.

Encouragement and New Strategies

Feeling supported by others who have faced similar challenges can be incredibly encouraging. It's comforting to know that setbacks are just part of the journey. Additionally, don't hesitate to experiment with advice or recipes from community members. While not everything will work for you, discovering new approaches is essential for engaging your fasting journey.

Mindful Eating Practices to Enhance Your Fasting Experience

Incorporating mindful eating into your daily routine transforms each meal into a chance to bond with your body and the nourishment it receives. This practice complements IF beautifully, forming a comprehensive approach to health that goes beyond just scheduling meals. Mindful eating is about immersing yourself in the current moment, focusing on the sensory experiences of eating—how the food smells, tastes, and feels. This can lead to a deeper appreciation of your meals and a more fulfilling dining experience.

The Principles of Mindful Eating

The essence of mindful eating is awareness. Notice the colors, textures, and tastes of your food. Be aware of your body's hunger and fullness signals, and observe your emotional reactions towards different foods. This helps you eat in response to physical hunger rather than emotional cravings, improving your digestion and creating a more rewarding relationship with food.

- **Awareness**: Check in with yourself before eating to see if you're starving or just eating out of habit.

- **Engagement**: When you're eating, engage your senses. Notice the details of each bite.

- **Response to Food**: Different foods make you feel physically and emotionally.

Eating Without Distraction

In our busy world, eating while distracted by screens or other activities is expected. To eat mindfully, try sitting at a table, turning off all electronic devices, and focusing solely on your meal. This helps with digestion by encouraging slower eating and thorough chewing, helps you better recognize when you're full and helps prevent overeating.

- **Environment**: Set up a peaceful, distraction-free area for eating.

- **Pace**: Slow down, put your utensil between bites, and chew well.

Savoring Every Bite

Treating each bite as a special moment can make meals more enjoyable and satisfying. Allow yourself to experience the flavors and textures of your food thoroughly. This approach can turn ordinary meals into delightful experiences.

- **Mindful Bites**: Try identifying the different flavors in your meal.

- **Gratitude**: Reflect on the effort and journey behind each dish, from the farmers to your preparations.

Gratitude for Food

Feeling thankful for your meals promotes a deeper connection with what you eat. It's about appreciating the journey from farm to plate and the nutrition your food provides. This sense of gratitude can make your eating experience more meaningful and mindful.

- **Sources**: Before eating, think about where your food came from and the effort that went into making it.

- **Nourishment**: Consider how the meal nourishes your body, giving you energy and health.

Blending mindful eating with IF elevates your eating from a mundane task to a profound, enriching experience. It fosters a healthier relationship with food characterized by gratitude, fulfillment, and attention to your body's needs. Adopting mindful eating principles enhances your fasting journey and overall well-being, making each meal a celebration of connection and joy.

Holistic Health: Viewing IF as Part of a Larger Picture

IF is more than just an eating schedule; it's a way to care for your body and mind, embracing every aspect of your well-being. This comprehensive approach to health means looking beyond your diet and considering how sleep quality, stress levels, and physical activity contribute to your overall condition. When you blend IF, with these other elements of health, you create a powerful combination that supports your body's natural rhythms and healing capabilities.

Beyond Just Dieting

Think of IF not as a solitary activity but as part of your broader health landscape. It interacts with crucial areas like sleep, stress management, and exercise, contributing to a well-rounded, healthy lifestyle. Fasting is most effective when it's part of a greater whole, working in harmony with other practices that enhance your overall well-being and help ward off chronic illnesses.

Integrative Wellness Practices

To make the most out of IF, you might want to include various wellness practices in your daily routine:

- **Yoga**: This can help stretch and strengthen your body while soothing your mind, reducing stress, and enhancing your sense of inner calm.

- **Meditation**: Regular meditation can improve mental clarity and reduce stress levels, sticking to your fasting schedule and making healthy eating choices more manageable.

- **Natural Therapies**: Consider trying therapies like acupuncture or massage to support your body's healing process and improve overall well-being.

- **Nature Walks**: Time spent outdoors can lower stress, boost your mood, and promote physical activity, all of which complement the benefits of IF.

Preventive Health

View IF as a preventive health strategy. It's not just about avoiding food for certain hours; it's about fostering your body's natural defenses against illness. IF can improve metabolism, reduce inflammation, and lower the risk of several chronic conditions, such as diabetes and heart disease. It is a potent preventative health tool that combines fasting with good sleep habits, stress management, and consistent exercise.

Continuous Learning

Health and wellness fields are constantly advancing, with new insights frequently emerging. Stay informed about the latest research and developments in IF and other wellness areas. Everyone's body is different; what works well for someone else may not suit you perfectly. By staying informed and flexible, you can adapt your approach to IF and overall health to meet your needs and goals.

Incorporating IF into a holistic health strategy allows you to look beyond food and fasting windows. It invites you to examine how all aspects of your life—diet, sleep, stress, and physical activity—interconnect to affect your health. Adopting this comprehensive viewpoint empowers you to make informed, balanced choices that support your body's needs, leading to a more balanced and vibrant life.

Adjusting Your Fasting Plan as Your Body and Goals Change

Our bodies and goals evolve as we go through life, and so should our approach to IF. It's all about creating a plan that aligns with our current needs and circumstances.

> *REAL JOURNEY: Anita, 50, found her rhythm with flexible fasting schedule after trying and struggling with more rigid methods. She allowed some leeway when fasting felt too challenging, opting for shorter fasting periods. This adaptation helped her maintain her routine without feeling overwhelmed. Anita learned that strict adherence wasn't as important as finding a sustainable, flexible approach that honored her body's needs.*

Listening to Your Body

Paying attention to your body is crucial. You might notice changes in how you feel with different fasting schedules or how certain foods affect you. If the 16/8 method you've been following no longer feels right—maybe you're feeling hungrier earlier or more tired—it's your body signaling it's time for a change.

- **Adjust Accordingly**: If you're feeling off, you might need to shorten your fasting window or adjust your eating to feel more satisfied.

- **Hydration and Sleep**: Monitor your hydration and sleep, too; changes here might indicate a need to tweak your fasting plan.

Evolving Health Goals

Your health goals might also shift over time. Perhaps you started fasting for weight loss but are more interested in metabolic health or longevity. This shift might be a time to reassess and adjust your fasting approach.

- **New Research and Methods**: Keep up with the latest IF and nutrition research. New information might lead you to modify your approach.

- **Goal-Specific Adjustments**: Tailor your fasting and diet to support your current health objectives, whether they're focused on blood sugar, energy levels, or something else.

Age-Related Adjustments

As we age, our bodies change, impacting how we respond to fasting. Metabolism, hormonal profiles, and physical activity levels all play a role.

- **Menopause and Andropause**: These stages of life come with hormonal changes that can affect your health and might necessitate changes to your fasting routine.

- **Physical Activity Levels**: If your activity levels change, your fasting and eating needs will likely change too.

Seeking Professional Guidance

Sometimes, making adjustments on your own isn't enough. If you're facing challenges with your fasting plan, have specific health conditions, or want personalized advice, it's a good idea to consult a professional.

- **Nutritionists and Dietitians**: They can provide customized guidance on your meals and nutritional needs to ensure your fasting plan fits your lifestyle and health status.

- **Medical Professionals**: If you have underlying health issues or are experiencing adverse effects from fasting, a healthcare provider can help determine the best course of action.

Adjusting your fasting plan as your life and body change is essential for maintaining its effectiveness and ensuring it continues to benefit you. Being open to modifications, listening to your body's signals, and seeking professional advice when necessary are all critical steps in keeping your fasting approach aligned with your current life stage and health goals.

Troubleshooting Common Challenges in IF

When practicing IF, facing challenges such as hunger pangs, energy dips, and social pressures is normal. These hurdles are common but can be managed with the right strategies, smoothing your fasting journey.

Identifying Common Fasting Challenges

Here's a look at some typical hurdles you might encounter:

- **Hunger Pangs**: This is not just about feeling hungry; it's also about the mental challenge it represents.

- **Energy Dips**: Sometimes, you might feel a drop in energy that makes you question your fasting schedule.

- **Social Pressures**: Questions or comments from others about your fasting can test your determination.

Strategies for Overcoming Challenges

For each of these challenges, there are effective ways to cope:

Managing Hunger Pangs:

REAL JOURNEY: Julia, 53, started IF to manage her weight and improve her energy levels. She chose the 16:8 method, fasting for 16 hours a day. Initially, Julia struggled with hunger pangs and headaches. However, she persisted, adjusting her eating window to better fit her lifestyle. Over six months, not only did she lose 15 pounds, but she also noticed improved mental clarity. Julia's success lies in her willingness to adapt and find what works best for her body.

- **Hydrate**: Drinking water can often quench what feels like hunger since our bodies can mix up hunger with thirst.

- **Stay Busy**: Distracting yourself with activities can help you ride out hunger pangs.

- **Low-Calorie Beverages**: Drinks like black coffee or herbal tea can help tide you over until your next meal.

Boosting Energy When It Dips:

- **Check Your Sleep**: Ensure you get enough rest, as lack of sleep can make fasting harder.

- **Review Your Diet**: Ensure your meals are balanced to maintain energy levels.

- **Move Around**: A short walk or light stretching can boost energy.

Navigating Social Pressures:

- **Prepare Your Responses**: Having ready answers to questions about your fasting can be helpful.

- **Suggest Non-Meal Activities**: Propose alternatives that don't revolve around eating, like walking or a non-meal get-together.

- **Explain Your Reasons**: Sharing why you're fasting may lead others to understand and respect your choices.

When to Break a Fast

It's important to know when to end a fast for your health's sake:

- **Feeling Unwell**: If you're dizzy, overly tired, or feeling off, it's time to eat something nutritious.

- **After Intense Physical Activity**: Replenishing your energy is essential if you've done a heavy workout.

- **Special Occasions**: Life is about balance. Don't hesitate to adjust your fasting for significant life events.

Adapting the Fasting Method

As your lifestyle or goals change, you might need to tweak your fasting approach:

- **Adjust Your Fasting Window**: If 16/8 is too challenging, try a shorter period like 14/10. Or, if you're comfortable, you might extend it.

- **Try Different Fasting Types**: If daily fasting is challenging, consider a method like 5:2, which involves less frequent fasting.

- **Shift Your Eating Window**: Align your eating times with your social life or energy needs, like changing your window to later in the day or starting earlier.

Using these strategies, you can adapt your fasting practice to fit your lifestyle and needs better. Remember, it's okay to adjust your approach as circumstances change; staying flexible is critical to maintaining your health and wellness goals while fasting.

Beyond Weight Loss: Monitoring Different Health Markers

IF is more than a tool for weight loss; it's a method that can significantly improve various aspects of your health. This approach to eating can influence everything from your metabolic function to your brain health and cellular resilience. It's important to understand that the body is a complex system, and changes in one aspect can profoundly affect your overall health.

Comprehensive Health Benefits

IF can lead to numerous health improvements. For instance, it can enhance metabolic health by improving insulin sensitivity and reducing blood sugar levels, which lowers the risk of type 2 diabetes and helps maintain steady energy throughout the day. Additionally, fasting boosts brain function by increasing the production of brain-derived neurotrophic factor (BDNF), enhancing memory and focus.

> *REAL JOURNEY: Ellen, 59 began IF with high hopes but faced significant setbacks. She often felt discouraged when the scale didn't reflect her efforts. But instead of giving up, Ellen focused on non-scale victories like more stable blood sugar levels, which were crucial for her as a diabetic. After a year of consistent effort, Ellen finally started seeing the weight loss she hoped for, teaching her the value of patience and consistency.*

On a cellular level, IF promotes autophagy, where cells cleanse themselves of damaged parts, leading to a healthier, more efficient system. This can help slow aging and reduce inflammation, contributing to a healthier, more vibrant body.

Monitoring Health Markers

To fully understand the effects of IF, it's important to monitor various health markers:

- **Blood Pressure**: Regular checks can reveal how fasting affects heart health.

- **Cholesterol Levels**: Observing changes in your cholesterol can provide insights into your cardiovascular health.

- **Blood Sugar Levels**: Especially important for those with diabetes or prediabetes, monitoring blood sugar can show the direct effects of fasting on metabolic health.

Including liver function tests and inflammatory markers like C-reactive protein in your monitoring can give a complete picture of the health benefits you're receiving from IF.

Personal Health Journeys

Everyone's experience with IF is unique. Journaling your fasting journey, including changes in your physical feelings, energy levels, and mental clarity, can offer valuable insights into how fasting impacts your life.

- **Energy and Alertness**: Note changes in your energy and mental sharpness to understand how your fasting schedule affects you.

- **Mood Fluctuations**: Tracking mood changes can help identify the emotional benefits of fasting, such as increased stability and reduced mood swings.

This personal record can motivate you and help refine your fasting approach to suit your needs and objectives better.

Consulting Healthcare Providers

Guidance from healthcare professionals is crucial when undertaking IF. They can ensure your fasting practices harmonize with your overall health and provide adjustments based on your health markers.

- **Preventative Screenings**: Regular health screenings can help identify and address potential issues early, allowing for timely adjustments to your fasting routine.

- **Personalized Advice**: A healthcare provider can offer tailored advice to ensure your fasting method is safe and effective.

Incorporating IF into your life is a journey towards a healthier, more fulfilling lifestyle. By recognizing its broad benefits, monitoring essential health markers, documenting your experiences, and seeking professional advice, you can ensure this practice contributes positively to your overall well-being, leading to a life that is not just longer but richer and more rewarding.

Maintaining Your New Lifestyle Long-Term

Adapting to IF as a part of your daily life is about creating a lifestyle that's uniquely yours and can evolve with you—viewing IF as a sustainable practice rather than a short-term diet can lead to meaningful, long-lasting changes. It's not just about weight loss—it's about how you feel overall, your engagement with the world, and nourishing both body and mind.

Long-Term Vision

Think of IF as a long-term partner in your health journey. It's essential to see how it aligns with your goals and aspirations. Focusing on the long-term benefits helps ensure that IF remains a positive influence in your life, adaptable and growing alongside you.

Continuous Adaptation

As your life changes, so should your approach to IF. Being open to adjusting your fasting schedule or dietary choices ensures the practice continues to meet your needs, no matter what changes come your way. This adaptability is crucial for making IF a valuable part of your life.

Celebrating Milestones

Recognize and celebrate every success along your fasting journey, big or small. Acknowledging these milestones reinforces the value of your efforts and keeps you motivated. Celebrate in meaningful ways—share with friends, indulge in a new experience, or reflect on how far you've come.

Inspiring Others

Your fasting journey can inspire others. By sharing your experiences, challenges, and successes, you can encourage others to improve their health. Share the holistic benefits you've experienced, including physical changes, mental clarity, and emotional well-being enhancements.

Looking Ahead

Remember, IF is just one part of a balanced lifestyle. Integrating it with nutritious eating, enjoyable physical activity, and other healthful habits creates a comprehensive approach to well-being that supports you through life's various stages.

In conclusion, adopting IF as a long-term lifestyle is more than following a schedule; it's about creating a life that fits your health goals and evolving needs. By maintaining a long-term perspective, staying flexible, celebrating your achievements, and sharing your journey, you set the foundation for a sustainable and enriching fasting experience that supports your well-being in every way.

Integrate Fasting with Ease

This framework is designed to help you integrate IF into your week smoothly and efficiently. Follow these prompts to plan, anticipate challenges, and ensure your fasting aligns with your lifestyle and commitments

MONDAY

Fasting Window: Identify your intended start and end times for fasting.

Potential Challenges: Note any specific challenges you might face today (e.g., a morning meeting with breakfast).

Meal Planning: Decide on your fasting-friendly meals for the day.

Adjustments: How will your schedule accommodate your fasting window?

Integrate Fasting with Ease

This framework is designed to help you integrate IF into your week smoothly and efficiently. Follow these prompts to plan, anticipate challenges, and ensure your fasting aligns with your lifestyle and commitments

TUESDAY

Fasting Window: Schedule your fasting period.

Potential Challenges: Anticipate any social or work-related events affecting your fasting.

Meal Planning: Outline your meals, focusing on nutrient-dense foods to break your fast.

Adjustments: Plan any necessary adjustments to your fasting window or meal times.

Integrate Fasting with Ease

This framework is designed to help you integrate IF into your week smoothly and efficiently. Follow these prompts to plan, anticipate challenges, and ensure your fasting aligns with your lifestyle and commitments

WEDNESDAY

Fasting Window: Confirm your fasting start and end times.

_____

_____

_____

_____

Potential Challenges: Identify midweek hurdles, like increased workload or social outings.

_____

_____

_____

_____

Meal Planning: Prepare a list of what you'll eat during your eating window.

_____

_____

_____

_____

Adjustments: Consider any tweaks to help you stay on track with fasting.

_____

_____

_____

_____

Integrate Fasting with Ease

This framework is designed to help you integrate IF into your week smoothly and efficiently. Follow these prompts to plan, anticipate challenges, and ensure your fasting aligns with your lifestyle and commitments

THURSDAY

Fasting Window: Look in your fasting times.

Potential Challenges: Look out for late-week challenges like dinner invitations.

Meal Planning: Plan your meals, perhaps introducing new recipes to keep things interesting.

Adjustments: Adjust your fasting window if you anticipate a late dinner or event.

Integrate Fasting with Ease

This framework is designed to help you integrate IF into your week smoothly and efficiently. Follow these prompts to plan, anticipate challenges, and ensure your fasting aligns with your lifestyle and commitments

FRIDAY

Fasting Window: Decide on your fasting period, possibly adjusting for weekend plans.

Potential Challenges: Friday social events or the temptation to unwind and snack.

Meal Planning: Choose meals that satisfy and sustain you through social activities.

Adjustments: Make any necessary modifications to your fasting schedule to enjoy your Friday.

Integrate Fasting with Ease

This framework is designed to help you integrate IF into your week smoothly and efficiently. Follow these prompts to plan, anticipate challenges, and ensure your fasting aligns with your lifestyle and commitments

SATURDAY

Fasting Window: Set a flexible fasting window for weekend leisure activities.

Potential Challenges: Weekend errands or family commitments that could disrupt your fasting routine.

Meal Planning: Plan a mix of quick, nutritious meals and possibly a meal out.

Adjustments: Be ready to adapt your fasting window based on weekend plans.

Integrate Fasting with Ease

This framework is designed to help you integrate IF into your week smoothly and efficiently. Follow these prompts to plan, anticipate challenges, and ensure your fasting aligns with your lifestyle and commitments

SUNDAY

Fasting Window: Plan a restful fasting period, preparing for the week ahead.

_____

_____

_____

_____

Potential Challenges: The temptation to end the week with a late-night snack.

_____

_____

_____

_____

Meal Planning: Prepare a wholesome dinner that sets you up for a successful fast start into the new week.

_____

_____

_____

_____

Adjustments: Reflect on the past week's successes and challenges to improve your IF integration.

_____

_____

_____

_____

Integrate Fasting with Ease

This framework is designed to help you integrate IF into your week smoothly and efficiently. Follow these prompts to plan, anticipate challenges, and ensure your fasting aligns with your lifestyle and commitments

WEEKLY REFLECTION

Successes: What went well? Celebrate your achievements.

Challenges: What obstacles did you face, and how did you overcome them?

Learnings: What did you learn about your body, habits, and preferences?

Adjustments for Next Week: Based on your experiences, how will you adjust your fasting plan for the next week?

Conclusion

"Your body hears everything your mind says. Stay positive, work hard, make it happen."

Anonymous

For women over 50, adopting IF is not just about starting a new diet; it's a step towards taking back control of your health, discovering a new source of vitality, and embracing life's changes with courage and poise. Solid science and your dedication have illuminated this journey, revealing the incredible empowerment and health improvements that come from a well-adjusted approach to IF.

The key insights from our journey rest on solid scientific evidence. IF's credibility for women after 50 is grounded in well-researched facts, not fads. This evidence confirms the effectiveness of IF and emphasizes the need for a personalized approach, acknowledging the unique challenges and demands of aging women.

The journey ahead is clear: Engage with an open heart and a well-informed mind with IF. Use scientific insights as your guide while paying close attention to your body's signals. Start with small changes, have patience, and be willing to adapt based on your experiences and what feels suitable for you.

In the dynamic health and wellness world, staying informed cannot be overstressed. Keep up with the latest in IF and health research. Embrace new information and be ready to adjust your lifestyle accordingly. This book is meant to be the first step on your path to better health, not the last.

Writing this book has been a shared journey of discovery. I hope the insights illuminate your way to a healthier, more fulfilling future. I am deeply thankful for your commitment to your health and for letting me be part of your journey to a vibrant life beyond 50.

Looking forward, I leave you with hope and encouragement. Remember, age is just a number, and adopting IF can unlock new potential for health and vitality. It's about making each moment richer, not just adding years to life.

As you move on from this book, I urge you to take practical steps to incorporate these lessons into your daily life. Seek reliable information on IF and women's health, utilize meal planning aids, and connect with fasting support communities to exchange stories and support.

Consider this book your guide to a future filled with wellness and joy. The journey of a thousand miles begins with a single step, and you've already taken that first stride. Here's to the road ahead, paved with discovery, health, and joy.

References

1. Dr. Brighten. (n.d.). Intermittent Fasting for Menopause: What You Need to Know. Retrieved from https://drbrighten.com/intermittent-fasting-for-menopause/

2. National Center for Biotechnology Information. (2021). Effect of Intermittent Fasting on Reproductive Hormone Levels in Women with Obesity: Results of a Randomized-Controlled Trial. Retrieved from https://www.ncbi.nlm.nih.gov/pmc/articles/PMC9182756/

3. Nature Aging. (2021). Autophagy in healthy aging and disease. Nature Aging, 1(1), 4-10. https://doi.org/10.1038/s43587-021-00098-4

4. Healthline. (n.d.). The Definitive Guide to Healthy Eating in Your 50s and 60s. Retrieved from https://www.healthline.com/nutrition/healthy-eating-50s-60s

5. Menopause Centre Australia. (n.d.). Intermittent Fasting During Menopause: What Do You Need to Know? Retrieved from https://www.menopausecentre.com.au/information-centre/articles/intermittent-fasting-during-menopause-what-do-you-need-to-know/

6. National Center for Biotechnology Information. (2021). Anti-Inflammatory Properties of Diet: Role in Healthy Aging. Retrieved from https://www.ncbi.nlm.nih.gov/pmc/articles/PMC8389628/

7. National Center for Biotechnology Information. (2021). Protein

Source and Muscle Health in Older Adults. Retrieved from https://www.ncbi.nlm.nih.gov/pmc/articles/PMC7996767/

8. National Institute on Aging. (n.d.). How can strength training build healthier bodies as we age? Retrieved from

9. Medical News Today. (n.d.). Intermittent fasting and exercise: How to do it safely. Retrieved from https://www.medicalnewstoday.com/articles/intermittent-fasting-and-working-out/

10. National Center for Biotechnology Information. (2012). Effectiveness of Yoga for Menopausal Symptoms. Retrieved from https://www.ncbi.nlm.nih.gov/pmc/articles/PMC3524799/

11. National Institute on Aging. (n.d.). Staying motivated to exercise: Tips for older adults. Retrieved from https://www.nia.nih.gov/health/exercise-and-physical-activity/staying-motivated-exercise-tips-older-adults

12. WebMD. (n.d.). What to know about intermittent fasting for women after 50. Retrieved from https://www.webmd.com/healthy-aging/what-to-know-about-intermittent-fasting-for-women-after-50

13. Longevity Technology. (n.d.). How to successfully adapt fasting into your lifestyle. Retrieved from https://longevity.technology/lifestyle/how-to-successfully-adapt-fasting-into-your-lifestyle/

14. Harvard T.H. Chan School of Public Health. (n.d.). Mindful eating. Retrieved from

15. National Center for Biotechnology Information. (2019). Effectiveness of Intermittent Fasting and Time-Restricted Feeding Compared to Continuous Energy Restriction for Weight Loss. Retrieved from https://www.ncbi.nlm.nih.gov/pmc/articles/PMC6836017/

We Appreciate Your Feedback

Keep the Game Alive!

"You have not lived today until you have done something for someone who can never repay you." - John Bunyan.

Now you have everything you need to embrace intermittent fasting for women over 50, it's time to pass on your newfound knowledge and show other readers where they can find the same help.

Simply by leaving your honest opinion of this book on Amazon, you'll show other women over 50 where they can find the information they're looking for and pass their passion for intermittent fasting forward.

Thank you for your help. The journey of intermittent fasting for women over 50 is kept alive when we pass on our knowledge – and you're helping us to do just that.

Simply click the link or scan the QR code below to leave your review:

https://www.amazon.com/review/review-your-purchases/?asin=B0D2WCLKXG

Leave a review

Thanks for being awesome!
Harmony Swift

Printed in Great Britain
by Amazon